Rare Disorders
That Cause Dysphagia

A GUIDE FOR SPEECH-LANGUAGE PATHOLOGISTS

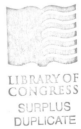

Rare Disorders That Cause Dysphagia

A GUIDE FOR SPEECH-LANGUAGE PATHOLOGISTS

Violet O. Cox, PhD, MLS, CCC-SLP

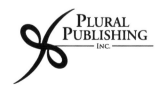

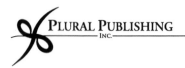

5521 Ruffin Road
San Diego, CA 92123

e-mail: information@pluralpublishing.com
Web site: https://www.pluralpublishing.com

Library of Congress Cataloging-in-Publication Data:

Names: Cox, Violet O., author.
Title: Rare disorders that cause dysphagia : a guide for speech-language
    pathologists / Violet O. Cox.
Description: San Diego, CA : Plural Publishing, Inc., [2020] | Includes
    bibliographical references and index.
Identifiers: LCCN 2019047169 | ISBN 9781635501421 (paperback) |
    ISBN 1635501423 (paperback) | ISBN 9781635501445 (ebook)
Subjects: MESH: Deglutition Disorders | Rare Diseases | Speech-Language
    Pathology—methods
Classification: LCC RC815.2 | NLM WI 258 | DDC 616.3/23—dc23
LC record available at https://lccn.loc.gov/2019047169

Contents

Introduction: Overview
of Rare Diseases

Rare diseases, whether in adults or children, have received increased attention over the last several years. This is most likely due to factors such as (1) increased public awareness from exposure to the internet, (2) improvement in the understanding and treatment of more common diseases, and (3) development of laws related to the treatment of rare medical conditions.

To date, there is no single definition of a rare disease, but there are at least three broadly accepted methods of defining rare diseases. Some of these definitions rely mainly on (1) the number of individuals surviving with the disease, (2) the availability of treatments for the disease, and (3) the severity of the disease.

In the United States, the Orphan Drug Act of 1983 (PL-97-414), created by Congress, defines a rare disease as any disease or condition which occurs infrequently. Later, the Rare Disease Act of 2002, which was based on the 1983 Orphan Drug Act, specifically defined a rare disease as "those which affect small patient populations, typically populations smaller than 200,000 individuals in the United States," or roughly 1 in 1,500 individuals (Genetics Home Reference, 2017). Initially, in the United States, the term "rare diseases" was categorized as "orphan diseases" largely because they did not offer a lucrative market for drug companies. However, the attitude of drug companies later changed with the enactment of the Orphan Drug Act that offered them financial incentives to develop new drugs to treat rare diseases.

Rare diseases are not limited to one country or region. They affect all countries of the world. In the country of Japan, a rare disease is legally defined as one that affects less than 50,000 individuals or 4 in 10,000. In Italy, there is no stated definition of a rare disease, but different measures have been used by various health institutions to categorize a disease as rare. For example, the Italian National Health Plan varies in its definition from 1 in 20,000 to 1 in 200,000. Countries that comprise the European Union (more than 30 countries) define a disease as rare if it affects fewer than 1 individual in 2,000. In these countries, more than 30,000,000 may be affected by at least one of the existing 7,000 rare diseases.

The National Center for Advancing Translational Sciences (NCATS) estimates that there are about 7,000 rare diseases with a further estimate of 25 million people living in the United States with one of these rare diseases and an estimated 30 million in Europe. This highlights the fact that while the disease may be rare, there is a disproportionately large number of individuals who continue to survive with the disease. One of the most difficult conundrums is that most of the rare diseases present with a wide range of underlying symptoms and disorders that vary from disease to disease and from patient to patient. This is further compounded by the fact that many ubiquitous symptoms can camouflage rare diseases, thus leading to a misdiagnosis of the disease, and hence a delay of appropriate treatment, and not surprisingly, the emergence of further sequelae of psychosocial ills and even morbidity. Of the many challenges diagnosticians face, the paucity of medical and scientific information about these diseases appears to be the most impactful, because it leads to a reduction in timely diagnosis and intervention.

Challenges

Physicians and the general medical community are extremely challenged by the field of rare diseases as evidenced by the long delay and missteps associated with diagnoses (Svenstrup, 2015). Recognizing and treating rare diseases create a further challenge to the medical profession in that 80% of these rare diseases are relatively few in number and spread out geographically, thus suffering from lack of research and limited expertise (United States Department of Health and Human Services, Public Health Service, Office of the Assistant Secretary for Health, 1989).

Many of the rare diseases identified carry common disorders—such as dysphagia and cognitive deficits—that require diagnosis and treatment provided by a speech-language pathologist. As its nomenclature readily suggests, a rare disease is infrequently seen by the physician and, not surprisingly, by other health-care specialists such as speech-language pathologists, physical therapists, and occupational therapists. The trickle-down effect here is that in the realm of common diseases, health-care specialists receive the referral from the physician to treat the patient, thus intervention occurs timely; but in the case of a rare disease, if the individual is not seen by the physician, then no referral can be made. On the other hand, most speech-language pathologists are familiar with common neurological diseases that cause swallowing disorders and a plethora of speech and language disorders and can readily diagnose and treat most of the speech and swallowing deficits. But in the case of a rare disease in which dysphagia is part of the symptomatology, lack of familiarity with the disease may fail to trigger a timely referral for speech intervention and most likely lead toward a much later intervention process. In attempting to unravel these challenges, it is probably a good idea to discuss dysphagia, which will be the center of the discussion throughout this book.

Dysphagia

Swallowing under normal circumstances is carried out with relatively little effort, yet it is a complex function. It is a process whereby masticated food, liquid, or saliva is forwarded through the mouth and finally to the stomach. Dysphagia is a common medical term used to describe a disorder of or difficulty with this transference of the food to the stomach. Based on the Taber's Cyclopedic Medical Dictionary, dysphagia can be classified into five subcategories (Groher & Crary, 2016):

1. Constricta dysphagia—disorder of swallowing due to narrowing of the pharynx or the esophagus

2. Lusoria dysphagia—swallowing disorder that arises from the compression of the esophagus by the right subclavian artery

3. Oropharyngeal dysphagia—difficulty transferring food from the mouth to the pharynx and esophagus

4. Paralytica dysphagia—swallowing disorder due to paralysis of the muscles of the mouth, pharynx, or esophagus

5. Spastica dysphagia—swallowing disorder that arises from spasms of the pharynx or esophagus

While dysphagia for the most part may not be a primary medical diagnosis, it is usually a strong symptom of an underlying medical condition, whether acquired or congenital. Its clinical symptoms can include coughing and/or choking during, after, or before swallowing; food sticking anywhere along the swallowing tract; regurgitation of food material; painful swallowing; drooling; and unexplained weight loss or nutritional deficiencies (Groher & Crary, 2016). There are a wide sequelae of physical, emotional, and psychosocial consequences that accompany dysphagia. Aspiration pneumonia, malnutrition, increased mortality, prolonged hospitalization, advanced disability, declined quality of life, and social isolation are but a few of the consequences of dysphagia (Eyigor 2013).

Prevalence of Dysphagia

Dysphagia can result from a myriad of specific disorders and categories of disorders, most of which are well-known to speech-language pathologists who routinely treat the swallowing problem. There is a wide variety of common neurological diseases associated with dysphagia. However, it is difficult to be precise in terms of the exact number of cases of dysphagia by disease or condition, but there are numerous reports that provide acceptable estimates. For example, dysphagia associated with strokes has been well docu-

Table 1. Classification of Some Common Conditions That May Cause Dysphagia

Classification	Conditions
Neurologic	Stroke, Parkinson's disease, multiple sclerosis, dementia, motor neuron diseases, myasthenia gravis, brain tumors
Myopathies	Endocrine myopathies, congenital myopathies, etc.
Rheumatologic	Sclerodoma, Sjogren's syndrome, dermatomyositis, polymyositis
Iatrogenic	Intubations/tracheostomy, neck surgery, medications, chemotherapy/radiation
Other	Respiratory disorders, congestive obstructive pulmonary disease

mented. Some disease states that are commonly associated with dysphagia are neurological, congenital, developmental, obstructions, muscular disorders, rheumatological disorders, as well as other nonspecific causes (Table 1).

Dysphagia is a relatively common and increasingly prevalent clinical problem. Estimated reports suggest that close to 10 million individuals in the United States are evaluated annually for some aspect of dysphagia. According to Bhattacharyya (2014), approximately 1 in 25 adults in the United States will experience some type of swallowing problem. Furthermore, about 22% of adults in primary care settings and 13.5% of the general population have some form of dysphagia. In addition, of those in the primary care setting who suffer with dysphagia, 80% are most likely to be females and 20% male (Wilkins, Gillies, Thomas, & Wagner, 2007). In spite of these numerical approximations, actual estimates of the prevalence of dysphagia is problematic for two basic reasons: (1) dysphagia can result from a multiplicity of diseases—both common and rare, and (2) it can affect both the young and elderly. Thus, it is not surprising that there are many underreported incidences of dysphagia. Nevertheless, a plethora of published reports substantiates the prevalence of dysphagia in older individuals. Schindler and Kelly (2002) reported that persons 65 years and older account for two-thirds of the individuals with dysphagia. According to data released by the U.S. Census Bureau, in April 2010 the total U.S. population increased by 9.7% and the number of persons age 65 years and older increased by 14.9% (U.S. Census Bureau, 2010). The census projected that for the next 18 years, 10,000 more Americans will become seniors each day; a natural phenomenon because of the aging baby boomer population. It is expected that by 2030, 1 in 5 U.S. residents will be 65 years of age or older.

Many studies (Cook, 2009; Marik & Kaplan, 2003; Rofes et al., 2010) have reported the presence of dysphagia in 50% of nursing home patients, with an increased risk of aspiration pneumonia and other complications more so in the elderly than in younger patients. However, it must be pointed out that aging does not cause dysphagia, but because the aging process is associated with measurable changes in neuromuscular activities, the risk for dysphagia is maximized in this population (Carucci & Turner, 2015). It has long been established that physiological deterioration is a hallmark of aging; however, it is not known how much of this deterioration is due to age or how much is due to age-related diseases and lifestyle. For example, in normal aging, there is cerebral atrophy, nerve function deterioration, and region-dependent decline in muscle mass that may influence swallowing (Masoro, 1987). Humbert and Robbins (2008) made an interesting distinction between "normal healthy aging swallow"—presbyphagia—and an otherwise disordered swallow—dysphagia. Presbyphagia has to do with characteristic changes that occur in the swallow mechanism in older individuals who are healthy (Robbins, Hamilton, Lof, & Kempster, 1992). Clinicians are becoming much more aware of these distinctions within the scheme of swallowing and are now able to make appropriate diagnoses. Added to this increased awareness is the fact that common conditions that precipitate dysphagia are well known to speech-language pathologists (see Table 1). These etiologies are routinely addressed in various textbooks on dysphagia.

In recent decades, there has been a burgeoning of medical information that has led to the identification of hitherto unknown diseases that carry sequelae of medical conditions including dysphagia. Given the rarity of these diseases, it is not surprising that many practicing speech-language pathologists are unaware of their existence. There is no question that knowledge of the etiology of dysphagia can inform intervention. Therefore, the purpose of this book is to identify and unpack rare diseases that are contributory to dysphagia in an easy and readily accessible form for the medical speech-language pathologist.

The next several chapters of this text will highlight a variety of rare diseases as identified by the National Organization of Rare Diseases (NORD) and the Genetic and Rare Diseases (GARD) information center. Of the more than 7,000 identified rare diseases in the world, the number that precipitate dysphagia is still largely unknown. However, through the National Institutes of Health (NIH), the Office of Rare Diseases Research (ORDR), as well as GARD, more information is surfacing as to the incidence of dysphagia in these diseases. Each chapter of this text has been divided into six sections aimed at providing a definition of the disease, history, causes (etiology), epidemiology, clinical manifestations/presentations, and diagnosis and treatment/management of the presenting dysphagia. One of the many "leaps" taken in writing this book is an attempt to quantify the epidemiological considerations of each type of rare disease.

Epidemiology deals with the incidence, prevalence/distribution, possible control of a disease, and other factors related to health. It is generally understood in the field of epidemiology that prevalence and incidence provide different measures about the occurrence of a disease. The *prevalence* of a condition means the number of persons with that condition, while *incidence* refers to the number of annually reported cases of the condition. But these two types of data reporting are fraught with inherent difficulties.

Prevalence data can be problematic for a number of reasons. First, there is no single method of quantifying data. For example, some prevalence data provide estimates on the number of actual diagnosed cases, while others include cases where individuals may be undiagnosed but may have symptoms of the disease. Secondly, the method of data collection can be inherently problematic as well. Some data may be obtained by a phone survey, while others may be obtained through other channels of research. A third problem that is present in prevalence data has to do with the "remission" or "cured" condition of the disease. Conditions that go into "remission" but are not necessarily "cured," such as cancer, have the potential to create problems for prevalence data. Some of these may use a 5-year or 10-year prevalence estimate. This then includes only people who have had cancer 5 or 10 years previously (even if they are "cured"). Thus, the assumption may be made that a remission becomes a cure after 5 or 10 years, so the person is then excluded from the prevalence numbers.

Incidence data, similar to prevalence data, are susceptible to problems. Incidence data measure the number of people who become affected with a condition each year, thus only new conditions, not ongoing treatment of existing conditions, are to be included. However, the actual number of people affected by a condition in a year may turn out to be less than stated in the incidence reports in cases where people get multiple cases of a condition. Since there is no one uniform method of reporting data, some incidence data may use government notifications or other various methods, or may be based on physician or hospital diagnoses. Nevertheless, in spite of the inherent problems that are encountered in epidemiological data, enough accurate information is still provided whereby appropriate interventions and management can be provided in each situation by medical personnel.

While this book targets medical speech-language pathologists as the main audience, the content is presented with just enough medical pedagogy to serve as a quick reference resource for physicians and other health-care providers.

References

Bhattacharyya, N. (2014). The prevalence of dysphagia among adults in the United States. *Otolaryngology-Head and Neck Surgery, 151*, 765–769.

Carucci, L. R., & Turner, M. A. (2015). Dysphagia revisited: Common and unusual causes. *Radiographics, 35*(1), 105–122.

Cook, I. J. (2009). Oropharyngeal dysphagia. *Gastroenterology Clinics, 38*(3), 411–431.

Eyigor, S. (2013). Dysphagia in rheumatological disorders. *World Journal of Rheumatology, 3*(3), 45–50.

Genetics Home Reference. (2017). FAQs about Rare Diseases. Retrieved from https://rarediseases.info.nih.gov/diseases/pages/31/faqs-about-rare-diseases

Groher, M. E., & Crary, M. A. (2016). *Dysphagia: Clinical management in adults and children.* St. Louis, MO: Elsevier Health Sciences.

Humbert, I. A., & Robbins, J. (2008). Dysphagia in the elderly. *Physical Medicine and Rehabilitation Clinics of North America, 19*(4), 853–866.

Marik, P. E., & Kaplan, D. (2003). Aspiration pneumonia and dysphagia in the elderly. *Chest, 124*(1), 328–336.

Masoro, E. J. (1987). Biology of aging. Current state of knowledge. *Archives of Internal Medicine, 147*(1), 166–169.

Robbins, J., Hamilton, J. W., Lof, G. L., & Kempster, G. B. (1992). Oropharyngeal swallowing in normal adults of different ages. *Gastroenterology, 103*(3), 823–829.

Rofes, L., Arreola, V., Romea, M., Palomera, E., Almirall, J., Cabré, M., . . . Clavé, P. (2010). Pathophysiology of oropharyngeal dysphagia in the frail elderly. *Neurogastroenterology & Motility, 22*(8), 851– 858.

Schindler, J. S., & Kelly, J. H. (2002). Swallowing disorders in the elderly. *Laryngoscope, 112*(4), 589–602.

Svenstrup, J. (2015). Rare disease diagnosis: A review of we search, social media and large-scale data mining. *Rare Diseases, 3*(1).

United States Department of Health and Human Services, Public Health Service, Office of the Assistant Secretary for Health. (1989). *Report of the National Commission on Orphan Diseases.* Rockville, MD: Author.

U.S. Census Bureau (2010, April 1). *Population and Housing Unit Counts* (REPORT NUMBER CPH-2). Retrieved from https://www2.census.gov/library/publications/decennial/2010/cph-2/cph-2-1.pdf

Wilkins, T., Gillies, R. A., Thomas, A. M., & Wagner, P. J. (2007). The prevalence of dysphagia in primary care patients: A HamesNet Research Network study. *Journal of the American Board of Family Medicine, 20*(2), 144–150.

Acknowledgments

The conceptualization of this volume from start to finish is largely due to the talents and encouragement of many individuals. First and foremost, I would like to acknowledge and thank Dr. Tony Sahley for his advice and support as well as Dr. Myrita Wilhite who facilitated this process through her wisdom and encouragement.

I am especially grateful to my graduate assistant McKenzie Witzke for her untiring reading of and commenting on portions of this text, as well as for her technological skills in editing the raw manuscript! Thanks also to the students in my neurogenic classes for their input in the selection of the cover for this book.

Finally, I want to thank the staff of Plural Publishing, especially Elisa Andersen for her invaluable assistance, as well as Kalie Koscielak and Valerie Johns for their patience.

—VC

Reviewers

Plural Publishing, Inc. and the author would like to thank the following reviewers for taking the time to provide their valuable feedback during the development process:

María A. Centeno, CCC-SLP, BCS-S
Universidad del Turabo

Vicki Hammen, PhD, CCC-SLP
Indiana State University

Amber Heape, ClinScD, CCC-SLP, CDP
PruittHealth Therapy Services
South Carolina State University
Rocky Mountain University of Health Professions

Michaela A. Medved, MA, TSSLD, CCC-SLP, ClinScD
Yeshiva University

Danielle R. Osmelak, EdD, CCC-SLP
Governors State University

Shannon Salley, SLPD, CCC-SLP
Coordinator, SLP Online
Longwood University

Dedicated to my daughter, Lee-Amor.

1

Plummer-Vinson Syndrome

> **KEY WORDS:** iron deficiency anemia, laryngeal webbing, sideropenia, phenotype, angular cheilitis, koilonychia, glossitis, esophageal webs

Definition

Plummer-Vinson syndrome (PVS), also known as Patterson-Brown-Kelly syndrome as well as sideropenic dysphagia, is listed as a rare disease by the Office of Rare Diseases (ORD) of the National Institutes of Health (NIH). Based on the definition of a rare disease, this means that PVS affects less than 200,000 persons in the United States. PVS falls within the categories of blood and digestive diseases. It is generally defined by its classic presentation of triad disorders. These are dysphagia, iron deficiency anemia, and laryngeal webbing. The main cause of the dysphagia is believed to be associated with the presence of a web in the cervical esophagus (Figure 1–1). Abnormal motility of the pharynx and the esophagus is also implicated (Lichtenstein, 1994; Plummer, 1912). The swallowing difficulties prominent in PVS are highly correlated with the small, thin growths of tissue—webbing—that tend to block the upper esophagus. However, while the pathogenesis of PVS is still largely unknown,

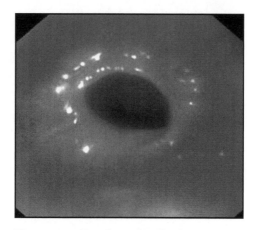

Figure 1–1. Esophageal web. *Source*: From "Recurrent multiple cervical esophageal webs: An unusual presentation of celiac disease," by U. Dutta, A. Khaliq, M. T. Noor, R. Kochhar, and K. Singh, 2009, *Gastroenterology Research*, 2(6), 356–357. doi:10.4021/gr 2009.12.1325

according to early researchers, the most probable cause is the iron deficiency (Okamura, Tsutsumi, Inaki, & Mori, 1988). This may be because with an iron deficiency, the loss of iron-dependent enzymes causes degeneration of tissue, atrophy, and the eventual formation of webs that are frequently seen in the upper esophageal region (see Figure 1–1).

History

Plummer-Vinson syndrome is eponymically linked to two prominent physicians of the Mayo Clinic: Henry Stanley Plummer (1874–1936), an internist/endocrinologist and founding member of the clinic; and Porter Paisley Vinson (1890–1959), a surgeon (Ormerod, 1966). Plummer identified a number of patients with a history of iron deficiency anemia, dysphagia, and spasm of the upper esophagus in the absence of anatomic stenosis. Later,

Vinson corroborated Plummer's findings when he reported similar esophageal aberrations in patients with dysphagia.

Another name for the disorder is Paterson-Kelly syndrome, named after two British laryngologists: Donald Ross Paterson (1863–1939) and Adam Brown-Kelly (1866–1941). These physicians not only independently reported characteristics of the disease, but also were actually the first to describe the characteristic features of the syndrome (in Novacek, 2006). The nomenclature for the disorder changes depending on location. In the United States, it is referred to as Plummer-Vinson syndrome; whereas in the United Kingdom, it is commonly known as Paterson-Kelly syndrome (Slater, 1991). The term "sideropenic dysphagia" is sometimes used for the disorder simply because iron deficiency or **sideropenia** is a key factor in the syndrome.

Etiology

While the cause of PVS remains unclear, many researchers have linked iron and nutritional deficiencies as well as genetic factors to the root cause. This rare disorder, in many cases of the condition, is associated with cancers of the throat and the esophagus. The pervasive iron deficiency theory present in PVS has been met with some measure of speculation, even though most of the earlier reports of the disorder cited iron deficiency in the pathogenesis of esophageal webs and dysphagia in a majority of predisposed patients (Okamura, Tsutsumi, Inaki, & Mori, 1988). Nevertheless, it is worth noting that the improvement in dysphagia in many cases following iron therapy does provide evidence for some association between the iron deficiency and the dysphagia (Chisholm, 1974).

Other etiologic factors such as malnutrition, genetic predisposition, and autoimmune processes have been proposed. The latter is based on the association between Plummer-Vinson syndrome and certain autoimmune disorders such as celiac disease (which was the most frequently mentioned associated disease in the case reports published in recent years), thyroid disease, and rheumatoid arthritis (Novacek, 2006).

Epidemiology

Currently, there are no reliable data about the incidence and prevalence of PVS as the disorder is now considered very rare. However, in the early part of the 20th century, the disease was noted to be prevalent in most middle-aged Caucasian women, specifically in Northern European countries. Since the syndrome is so rare, only case reports as opposed to "series" of patient reports have been published in recent literature. The rarity of PVS appears to correlate with improvement in nutritional status, availability of health care, and the widespread addition of iron and iron-supplemented diets. Although PVS has been more frequently observed in females between 40 to 70 years of age, there have been a few reported incidences of the disorder in children as well as in males (Mansell, Jani & Bailey, 1999). Bakshi (2015) reported a high occurrence of PVS in India in both males and females. A review of the English language case reports published between 1999 and 2005 revealed that 25 out of 28 cases (89%) were females (Novacek, 2006) with a mean age of 47, ranging from 28 years of age to 80 years of age.

Clinical Presentation

It is well known medically that in most diseases, symptoms vary from person to person. Consequently, it is not surprising that people with the same disease may not manifest all of the known symptoms of the particular disease. The Human Phenotype Ontology foundry (HPO or HP) provides a standardized vocabulary of **phenotypic** abnormalities that are identified in human diseases. Various categories of HPO associations are linked to

PVS (Table 1–1). While most patients will not exhibit all of the symptoms established for PVS (Table 1–2), all of them will manifest the triad of dysphagia, iron deficiency, and an esophageal web (Figure 1–2).

Apart from the classic symptoms described above, there are a number of other presenting disorders commonly seen in PVS such as glossitis, angular cheilitis, and koilonychia.

Glossitis: The National Institutes of Health (NIH) defines glossitis as a general term for inflammation of the tongue. Of the many causes of glossitis, iron deficiency is recognized as a major contributor. Bayraktar and Bayraktar (2010) suggest that atrophy of the upper GI mucosa caused by iron deficiency leads to the inflammatory nature of the tongue. This condition is often characterized by depapillation of the dorsal aspects of the tongue. In some cases of glossitis, the tongue can become so swollen that chewing, swallowing, and speaking may be difficult.

Angular cheilitis: This inflammatory condition can affect one or both corners (angles) of the mouth. Typically, the condition is characterized by erythema (redness), cracked lips, and bleeding and ulcerated corners of the lips—all of which tend to cause pain. Angular cheilitis can result from many conditions such as fungus, bacteria, or malnutrition. In the case of malnutrition, angular cheilitis is most often caused by the iron deficiency anemia that is linked to PVS (Figure 1–3).

Koilonychia: A condition in which the fingernails present as thin with lifted outer edges, resembling the shape of a spoon, hence also known as "spoon nails." This condition is present in cases of iron deficiency or poor absorption of iron as in PVS.

As has been previously discussed, the diagnostic criteria for PVS feature dysphagia, esophageal webs, and iron deficiency anemia as the three key players (Skolka & Pauly-Hubbard, 2017). Of great interest is the interrelatedness of these three different symptoms that apparently must exist together in order to make

Table 1–1. Plummer-Vinson Human Phenotype Ontology
Associations (HP)

Head & Neck		
Term Identifier	**Name**	**Definition**
HP:0100825	Cheilitis	Inflammation of the lip
HP:0000160	Narrow mouth	Decreased width of oral aperture
HP:0000206	Glossitis	Inflammation of the tongue
HP:0012473	Tongue atrophy	Wasting of the muscles of the tongue
HP:0010284	Intraoral hyperpigmentation	Increased pigmentation of the oral mucosa either focal or generalized
Blood & Blood- Forming Tissues		
Term Identifier	**Name**	**Definition**
HP:0004840	Hypochromic micro-cytic anemia	A type of anemia characterized by an abnormally low concentration of hemoglobin in the erythrocytes and lower than normal size of the erythrocytes
HP:0001891	Iron deficiency anemia	

Table 1–1. *continued*

Digestive System		
Term Identifier	**Name**	**Definition**
HP:0100594	Esophageal web	Thin (2–3mm) membranes of normal esophageal tissue consisting of mucosa and submucosa that can be congenital or acquired. Congenital webs commonly appear in the middle and inferior third of the esophagus, and they are more likely to be circumferential with a central or eccentric orifice. Acquired webs are much more common than congenital webs and typically appear in the cervical area (postcricoid). Clinical symptoms of this condition are selective (solids more than liquids) dysphagia, thoracic pain, nasopharyngeal reflux, aspiration, perforation, and food impaction (the last two are very rare).
HP:0002015	Dysphagia	Difficulty swallowing

continues

Table 1–1. *continued*

Skin, Hair, and Nails		
Term Identifier	**Name**	**Definition**
HP:0000980	Pallor	Abnormally pale skin
HP:0001598	Concave nail	The natural longitudinal (posterodistal) convex arch is not present or is inverted

Metabolism/Laboratory Abnormality		
Term Identifier	**Name**	**Definition**
HP:0012343	Decreased serum ferritin	Abnormally reduced concentration of ferritin, an ubiquitous intracellular protein that stores iron in the blood

Nervous System		
Term Identifier	**Name**	**Definition**
HP:0003388	Easy fatigability	Increased susceptibility to fatigue

Constitutional Symptom		
Term Identifier	**Name**	**Definition**
HP:0002027	Abdominal	An unpleasant sensation characterized by physical discomfort (such as pricking, throbbing, or aching) and perceived to originate in the abdomen

Source: Adapted from "The human phenotype ontology in 2017" by S. Köhler, N. A. Vasilevsky, M. Engelstad, E. Foster, J. McMurry, S. Aymé, . . . P. N. Robinson, 2017, *Nucleic Acids Research*, 45, D865–D876.

Table 1–2. Clinical Symptoms in Plummer-Vinson

Clinical Symptoms
Present in All Cases of Pvs
Decreased serum ferritin
Dysphagia
Esophageal web
Hypochromic microcytic anemia
Iron deficiency anemia
Present in 80%–99% Cases of PVS
Easy fatigability
Glossitis
Pallor
Present in 5%–29% Cases of PVS
Abdominal pain
Cheilitis
Concave nail
Intraoral hyperpigmentation
Narrow mouth
Tongue atrophy

the case for PVS. As it turns out, these three different symptoms may be more connected than originally thought. But the disorder is not limited to these three conditions. It seems as though other shadowy symptoms manifested in PVS are all linked to the big triad. For example, it is postulated that the esophageal webs prominent in PVS may be due to long-term iron deficiency anemia, and, consequently, the fatigue, weakness, and pallor that are present in

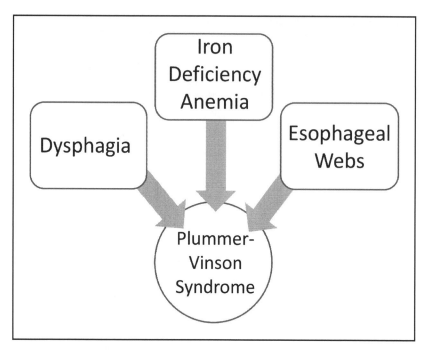

Figure 1–2. Triad of disorders in Plummer-Vinson syndrome. *Source*: From "Rare diseases that cause dysphagia: Plummer-Vinson syndrome," by V. O. Cox, 2018, *Journal of Phonetics & Audiology*, 4(1), 138. doi:10.4172/2471-9455.1000138

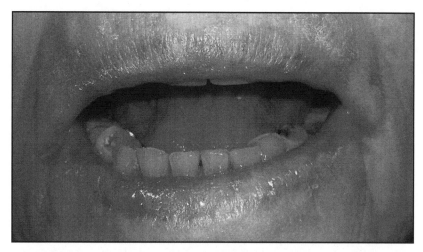

Figure 1–3. A photograph of angular cheilitis and glossitis. *Source*: File: Angular cheilitis1.jpg (2017, November 27). Wikimedia Commons, the free media repository. Retrieved 5 February 2019 from https://commons.wikimedia.org/w/index.php?title=File:Angular_cheilitis1.jpg&oldid=269449640.

individuals with PVS are all related to the classic anemia that can be routed back to iron deficiency, which eventually leads to the formation of these esophageal webs. In turn, the esophageal webs, which are thin mucosal folds that protrude into the lumen of the proximal esophagus, contribute to the classic dysphagia.

Dysphagia

Dysphagia is one of the main clinical features of Plummer-Vinson syndrome, but because there are many other causes of dysphagia, a differential diagnosis has to be made. The postcricoid dysphagia seen in PVS is also present in motility disorders such as achalasia as well as other disorders such as scleroderma, diabetes mellitus, gastroesophageal reflux disease (GERD), and most commonly in neurological and skeletal muscular disorders; therefore, these diseases must first be ruled out.

The nature of the dysphagia seen in individuals with PVS varies. In some patients, it has been described as painless, ranging from intermittent to progressive occurrence. Classically, most patients experience choking or fear of choking on specific food textures. Usually, these dysphagic symptoms tend to occur more so with solid textures. Typical, videofluoroscopic evaluation of the swallow may reveal delayed emptying of material in the hypopharyngeal region. Some patients may also experience a sudden onset of the dysphagia, but usually it tends to be insidious. It is not uncommon for patients to experience weight loss. This weight loss may be attributed to either avoidance of eating for fear of choking or compensatory changes in diet. The presence of the esophageal webs has reportedly caused choking spells and aspiration on solid foods in some patients, although others have experienced regurgitation on both solids and liquids (Skolka et al., 2017). Patients usually identify the neck area or above the suprasternal notch as the site of the obstruction when trying to explain the choking they experience.

Endoscopic studies have linked the manifestation of dysphagia to the size of the luminal diameter in the region of the esophageal web. Two independent studies suggest that in most patients with PVS, dysphagia should be graded in terms of the size of the luminal diameter, specifically, if the lumen is less than 12 mm. These studies described four levels of severity. Grade I, in which patients exhibiting difficulty swallowing solids was found in 52% of the cases. Grade II, in which patients who were only able to swallow semisolid foods was present in 36% of the cases. On the other hand, grade III dysphagia, in which the patients could only swallow liquids, and grade IV, in which patients had an inability to tolerate liquids was noted in 8% and 4%, respectively. These two latter levels appeared to be less common (Goel, Lakshmi, Bakshi, Soni, & Koshy, 2016; Sinha, Prajapati, George, & Gupta, 2006). Most cases of PVS confirm difficulty swallowing solid foods and in all cases, the dysphagia is associated with the presence of esophageal webs.

Esophageal Webs

Esophageal webs can be detected by a barium swallow X-ray, but the best way for demonstration is via videofluoroscopy (Chung & Roberts-Thomson, 1999). Esophageal webs are also detectable by upper gastrointestinal endoscopy. Visually, they appear smooth, thin, and gray. Webs typically occur in the proximal part of the esophagus and may be visually undetected or accidentally ruptured unless the endoscope is introduced under direct visualization (Hoffman & Jaffe, 1995). Esophageal webs can cause a feeling of chest pain in some patients with PVS. Typically, these patients may not associate the pain with dysphagia initially, as they may be continuing to consume food in their usual manner and mistaking the source of the pain to be unrelated to swallowing (Kuwabara & Tanaka, 2018). Webs are often located in the postcricoid region of the esophagus, which is a muscular tube that connects the pharynx with the stomach. It courses down posterior to the trachea and heart and just anterior to the spinal column. Because of its lengthy course, pain in the esophagus can often be mistaken for heartburn or indigestion.

Besides dysphagia and the presence of esophageal webs, another equally important element in the diagnosis of PVS is the presence of iron deficiency anemia. In fact, this is frequently the major discovery before dysphagia is identified.

Iron Deficiency Anemia

The presence of **iron deficiency anemia** (IDA) is part of PVS diagnosis. It is believed that IDA leads to rapid loss of iron-dependent enzymes due to its high cell turnover. Loss of these enzymes causes mucosal degenerations, atrophic changes, and web formation, which have been shown to lead to dysphagia (Okamura et al., 1988). This notion is supported by reports that the dysphagia in PVS tends to be relieved when the patient is treated with iron supplements (Sugiura, Nakagawa, Hashizume, Nemoto, & Kaseda, 2015; Tahara et al., 2014).

IDA is associated with other nutritional deficiencies in riboflavin, thiamine, and pyridoxine. Other complications linked to dysphagia that result from IDA are mucosal changes in the oropharynx such a stomatitis, atrophy of the lingual epithelium, depapillation, and angular cheilosis. Although frequent occurrences of dysphagia, hypopharyngeal, and oral cancers have been reported in some cases of IDA, these reports are still inconclusive (Goel, Bakshi, Soni, & Chhavi, 2017).

As mentioned earlier in this chapter, in diagnosing PVS from other causes of dysphagia, it is important to determine the cause of the dysphagia. The clinician has to bear in mind that causes of dysphagia other than PVS are common; therefore, these causes must be ruled out. Goel et al. (2017) identified a number of benign causes that result in esophageal dysphagia. Some of these are Zenker's diverticulm, esophageal strictures secondary to corrosive injury, or surgical anastomosis of the esophagus specifically after surgery to repair a tracheoesophageal fistula. Other esophageal motility disorders such as scleroderma or achalasia cardia are some causes of dysphagia in PVS.

Management of Dysphagia

In general, dysphagia in PVS has an excellent recovery outcome even though PVS is categorized as a precancerous condition. Patients with PVS are considered to be at risk for squamous cell carcinoma of the hypopharynx or upper esophageal region. The good news in treatment for many patients with PVS is that with treatment for IDA, the dysphagia as well as the esophageal webs tends to resolve over time (Sugiura et al., 2015; Tahara et al., 2015).

The usual symptoms of dysphagia secondary to PVS described by most patients are difficulty swallowing solids, sensation of discomfort, and tightness or fullness typically described in the neck or chest region. Management of this type dysphagia is never the sole responsibility of the speech-language pathologist (SLP), since the primary concern is to improve the IDA. The SLP, however, still plays a vital role in terms of recommending strategies for safe swallowing such as posturing techniques if indicated, adjusting bolus viscosity and size, having the patient alternate solid foods with liquids, and other compensatory strategies.

Management of the IDA in PVS has been closely linked to the successful improvement of dysphagia in the patient. Different modes of management have been described in the literature. One approach is to treat with iron supplements. Iron supplements have proven to improve the swallowing deficits experienced by most patients. IDA in the first place is caused by a lack of iron; therefore, anemia develops when there is not enough iron in the body for hemoglobin synthesis. The lack of iron causes myasthenic changes to occur in muscles that are involved in the swallowing mechanism. This muscle weakness causes atrophy of the esophageal mucosa and leads to the formation of webs. Thus, it makes sense to treat the iron deficiency in an effort to reverse the process that caused the web to occur in the first place and simultaneously eliminate or reduce the dysphagia. Not all webs respond to the iron therapy; denser webs may result in more severe esophageal dysphagia and may require a more aggressive management, such as the use of endoscopic dilatation (Samad, Mohan, Balaji, Augustine, & Patil, 2015).

Summary

PVS is an iron deficiency anemia that is associated with esophageal webs and dysphagia usually in women. Typically, patients complain of choking and/or fear of swallowing. Even though the dysphagia is usually painless, some patients have complained of odynophagia. Symptoms secondary to the iron deficiency, such as muscle weakness, tend to dominate the clinical presentation of PVS. While the etiopathogenesis of PVS is still unknown, iron deficiency anemia is paramount in the discovery of the disorder. PVS in most cases can be effectively managed with iron supplements and endoscopic dilatation. However, since patients with PVS are at an increased risk for squamous cell esophageal carcinoma, the medical team follows them closely.

References

Bakshi, S. S. (2015). Plummer-Vinson syndrome—Is it common in males? *Arquivos de Gastroenterologia*, *52*(3), 250–252.

Bayraktar, U. D., & Bayraktar, S. (2010). Treatment of iron deficiency anemia associated with gastrointestinal tract diseases. *World Journal of Gastroenterology*, *16*(22), 2720.

Chisholm, M. (1974). The association between webs, iron and post-cricoid carcinoma. *Postgraduate Medical Journal*, *50*(582), 215–219.

Chung, S., & Roberts-Thomson, I. C. (1999). Gastrointestinal: Upper oesophageal web. *Journal of Gastroenterology and Hepatology*, *14*(6), 611.

Cox, V. (2018). Rare diseases that cause dysphagia: Plummer-Vinson syndrome. *Journal of Phonetics & Audiology*, *4*(1), 138–144.

Dutta, U., Khaliq, A., Noor, M. T., Kochhar, R., & Singh, K. (2009). Recurrent multiple cervical esophageal webs: An unusual presentation of celiac disease. *Gastroenterology Research, 2*(6), 356–357. doi:10.4021 /gr2009.12.1325

Goel, A., Bakshi, S. S., Soni, N., & Chhavi, N. (2017). Iron deficiency anemia and Plummer–Vinson syndrome: Current insights. *Journal of Blood Medicine, 8,* 175.

Goel, A., Lakshmi, C. P., Bakshi, S. S., Soni, N., & Koshy, S. (2016). Single-center prospective study of Plummer-Vinson syndrome. *Diseases of the Esophagus, 29*(7), 837–841.

Hoffman, R. M., & Jaffe, P. E. (1995). Plummer-Vinson syndrome: A case report and literature review. *Archives of Internal Medicine, 155*(18), 2008–2011.

Köhler, S., Vasilevsky, N. A., Engelstad, M., Foster, E., McMurry, J., Aymé, S., . . . Robinson, P. N. (2017). The human phenotype ontology in 2017. *Nucleic Acids Research, 45,* D865–D876.

Kuwabara, M., & Tanaka, M. (2018). A web effect: Plummer-Vinson syndrome. *The American Journal of Medicine, 131*(5), 504–505.

Lichtenstein, G. R. (1994) Esophageal rings, webs, and diverticula. In W. S. Haubrich (Ed.) *Bockus gastroenterology,* Vol. 1 (5th ed., pp. 518–523). Philadelphia, PA: W. B. Saunders Company.

Mansell, N. J., Jani, P., & Bailey, C. M. (1999). Plummer-Vinson syndrome—A rare presentation in a child. *Journal of Laryngology & Otology, 113*(5), 475–476.

Novacek, G. (2006). Plummer-Vinson syndrome. *Orphanet Journal of Rare Diseases, 1*(1), 36.

Okamura, H., Tsutsumi, S., Inaki, S., & Mori, T. (1988). Esophageal web in Plummer-Vinson syndrome. *Laryngoscope, 98*(9), 994–998.

Ormerod, F. C. (1966). Plummer-Vinson or Paterson-Brown-Kelly priority, precedence or prestige? *Journal of Laryngology & Otology, 80*(9), 894–901.

Plummer, H. S. (1912). Diffuse dilatation of the esophagus without anatomic stenosis (cardiospasm): A report of ninety-one cases. *Journal of the American Medical Association, 58*(26), 2013–2015.

Samad, A., Mohan, N., Balaji, R. S., Augustine, D., & Patil, S. G. (2015). Oral manifestations of Plummer-Vinson syndrome: A classic report with literature review. *Journal of International Oral Health, 7*(3), 68.

Sinha, V., Prajapati, B., George, A., & Gupta, D. (2006). A case study of Plummer-Vinson syndrome. *Indian Journal of Otolaryngology and Head and Neck Surgery, 58*(4), 391–392.

Skolka, M., & Pauly-Hubbard, H. (2017). Rapidly progressive Plummer-Vinson syndrome. *Journal of Rare Disorders: Diagnosis & Therapy, 3,* 1–3.

Slater, S. D. (1991). The Brown Kelly-Paterson or Plummer-Vinson syndrome: An old score finally settled. *Journal of the Royal College of Physicians of London, 25*(3), 257.

Sugiura, Y., Nakagawa, M., Hashizume, T., Nemoto, E., & Kaseda, S. (2015). Iron supplementation improved dysphagia related to Plummer-Vinson syndrome. *Keio Journal of Medicine, 64*(3), 48–50.

Tahara, T., Shibata, T., Okubo, M., Yoshioka, D., Ishizuka, T., Sumi, K., & Arisawa, T. (2014). A case of Plummer-Vinson syndrome showing rapid improvement of dysphagia and esophageal web after two weeks of iron therapy. *Case Reports in Gastroenterology, 8*(2), 211–215.

2

Niemann-Pick Disease Type C

KEY WORDS: Niemann-Pick, autosomal recessive, lysosomal, hepatosplenomegaly, acid sphingomyelinase, sphingomyelin, ceramide, mutation

Definition

Niemann-Pick disease (NPD) is a rare, autosomal recessive, inherited disorder in the group of lysosomal storage diseases caused by genetic mutations that interfere with metabolism. In these inherited diseases, lipids collect in the cells of the body. Individuals with NPD experience symptoms related to progressive neurological disorders as well as other vital organs such as the spleen and the liver. While NPD can occur at any age, it mainly affects children and is fatal.

Among the cluster of NPDs, there are three common types: NPD types A, B, and C. Each type appears to affect different organs of the body and can cause different symptoms. NPD types A and B are classified as those with deficiency of acid sphingomyelinase activity. Some infants with type A usually show signs and symptoms as early as in the first few months of life. Those with type B may not exhibit signs for years and tend to have a better chance of achieving adulthood.

According to the National Organization for Rare Diseases (NORD), Niemann-Pick disease type C (NPC) is a rare, progressive genetic disorder characterized by an inability of the body to transport cholesterol and other fatty substances (lipids) inside of cells. This leads to the abnormal accumulation of these substances within various tissues of the body, including brain tissue. The accumulation of these substances damages the affected areas. NPC is highly variable and the age of onset and specific symptoms can vary from one person to another, sometimes even among members of the same family. NPC can range from a fatal disorder within the first few months after birth (neonatal period) to a late onset, chronic, progressive disorder that remains undiagnosed well into adulthood. Most cases are detected during childhood and progress to cause life-threatening complications by the second or third decade of life. NPC is caused by mutations in the NPC1 gene (NPC type 1C) or the NPC2 gene (NPC type 2C), and is inherited in an **autosomal recessive** manner. The NPC1 and NPC2 genes provide instructions for creating protein found within the lysosomes and endosomes of cells. The exact function of this protein is still unclear, but it is believed to be important for the transport of cholesterol and other lipids within cells as well as across cell membranes.

History

Niemann-Pick disease (NPD) was first described in 1914 by a German pediatrician, Albert Niemann who identified the case of an 18-month-old with **hepatosplenomegaly**. Hepatosplenomegaly is a medical condition in which both the liver and the spleen become enlarged. In addition to this disorder, Niemann identified progressive neurologic deterioration and postmortem evidence of lipid accumulation (Fink, 2004). Several years later, in the 1920s, Ludwig Pick, a German pathologist, analyzed postmortem tissues from children with clinical signs previously described by Niemann and was able to establish the disorder as a new and distinct disease. Subsequent to their collaborative work, the eponym Niemann-Pick disease has been used to designate a heterogeneous group of lipid storage disorders with and without neurological involvement (Vanier, 2010). The clinical classification of NPD was separated into four different subtypes (A, B, C, and D) by Crocker (1961) based on clinical and biochemical data. NPD types A and B (NPA and NPB) are caused by mutations in the sphingomyelin phosphodiesterase gene (SMPD1). The gene, SMPD1, provides instructions for making an enzyme called **acid sphingomyelinase (ASM)**. This enzyme is found in **lysosomes**, which are small compartments in the cell that digest and recycle molecules. Acid sphingomyelinase is responsible for the conversion of a fat (lipid) called **sphingomyelin** into another type of lipid called **ceramide**. Sphingomyelin also binds (attaches) to a fat called cholesterol and helps to form other lipids that play roles in various cell processes. The formations of these lipids are critical for the normal structure and function of cells and tissues. A deficiency in acid sphingomyelinase leads to a buildup of accumulation of sphingomyelin within the cells. Both NPA and NPB are classically defined by the onset and severity of the disease (Davidson & Walkley, 2010). Type A is typically seen in infants and is characterized by severe neurological deficits, and most of these infants rarely survive to the age of two. Type B on the other hand appears later in juveniles but with minimal neurological impairment. The third type of NPD referred to as type C (NPC) occurs when the body is unable to breakdown or metabolize the high amount of cholesterol and lipids accumulated within the body. This condition causes widespread systemic and neurologic disorders throughout the body.

Etiology

NPD results from mutations in the specific genes that are directly responsible for how the body metabolizes fat. The term "**mutation**" refers to a change in a gene that prevents it from functioning normally. In order for an individual to inherit NPD, both parents

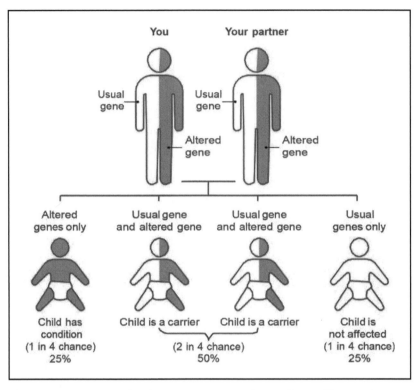

Figure 2–1. Autosomal inheritance pattern. *Source*: From "Improving outcomes for babies with genetic disorders," by Public Health England, 2015, September 18 (https://www.phescreening.blog.gov.uk/2015/09/18/improving-outcomes-for-babies-with-genetic-disorders/).

must be carriers of the defected gene that is passed on to the child (Figure 2–1). Genes constitute the blueprints for creating the proteins the body needs for development. Most genes come in pairs, one from each biological parent. A recessive gene produces an effect in the organism only when that gene is transmitted by both parents. Therefore, to inherit an autosomal disorder, both genes in a pair must be abnormal and each of the two genes must come from both biological parents who are the carriers of the defected gene. Carriers are usually not affected with the condition, even though they can pass the abnormal gene on to their offspring. Unfortunately, this is precisely the case in NPD in which the gene responsible for producing and metabolizing the essential lipids in the body are unable to perform their function.

As previously discussed, ASM is required to break down or metabolize the lipids in the body known as sphingomyelin. If there is a deficiency in ASM, sphingomyelin and other substances can accumulate in various tissues of the body. When sphingomyelin is not metabolized, it accumulates in organ tissue and causes substantial damage to the lungs, spleen, and liver as well as within the nervous system in severe cases. This condition interferes with the body's organs working smoothly and can be fatal. NPD types A and B, which result when there is an insufficient production of ASM, are caused by the same enzymatic deficiency, but they appear to represent opposite ends of a spectrum. Type A presents greater challenges to mortality. People with type A tend to have little to no production of ASM, while those with type B have approximately 10% of the normal production of ASM. Type A tends to have severe neurological deficits that lead to early death by 2 to 4 years of age. On the other hand, patients with type B show minimal neurological deficits, and may survive well in to adulthood but with other significant health complications such as enlarged livers and spleens that ultimately lead to cardiovascular disorders.

The third subtype of Niemann-Pick disease, type C (NPC), is the rarest and is much different from types A and B. Recall that in types A and B there is either not enough or absent ASM in the cells to remove the lipids; consequently, there is a buildup of these fats. In NPC, on the other hand, the body is not able to metabolize the cholesterol as well as the other lipids within the cell. Consequently, in type C, there are excessive amounts of cholesterol that accumulate in vital body organs such as the spleen, liver, and lungs as well as within the brain. Type C symptoms may appear as early as within a few months of life or well into adulthood. But there are a cacophony of health challenges, including dysphagia, that accompanies this type. It is important to understand the processes involved in NPC in order to appreciate the sequelae of disorders.

No two individuals with NPC will show the exact same characteristics. Sevin et al. (2007) carried out a comprehensive study of 68 patient with NPC and were able to identify the frequency of a number of major clinical, radiological, biochemical, and genotypic characteristics of the disease.

According to the National Organization for Rare Disorders (NORD), NPC belongs to a larger group of more than 50 disorders known as **lysosomal** storage disorders. Lysosomes are membrane-bound compartments within cells. They contain enzymes that break down larger molecules such as proteins, carbohydrates, and fats into their building blocks. Abnormal functioning of a transport protein can result in the accumulation of cholesterol and other fatty substances throughout the body including the brain. Because of the widespread buildup of cholesterol throughout the body, individuals with NPC present with an array of systemic and neurovascular disorders as well as psychiatric disorders. Clinically, the disease is heterogeneous and there is much variability from patient to patient. For the purposes of this chapter, greater discussions will center around NPD type C as opposed to types A and B. This is largely because dysphagia symptoms are manifested more so in NPC. Additionally, NPC covers a wider age range of disease onset.

Epidemiology

NPC including both the C1 and C2 types is a panethnic autosomal recessive inheritance disease. It is difficult to assess its true prevalence because of insufficient clinical assessment and the limitations in performing biochemical testing (Vanier, 2010). The clinical spectrum of this disease ranges from a neonatal, rapidly fatal disorder to an adult-onset, chronic, neurodegenerative disease (Sevin et al., 2007). Individuals with NPC can exhibit onset of symptoms at different ages that have been grouped historically as perinatal (shortly before or after birth), early infantile (3 months to less than 2 years), late infantile (2 years to less than 6 years), juvenile (6 to less than 15 years), and adult (15 years and older) (Genetic and Rare Disease Information Center, 2019).

Generally speaking, the life-span of patients can range from a few days until well into the fourth decade of life, although some studies have reported individuals reaching the sixth or seventh decades of life (Trendelenburg et al., 2006; Vanier, 2010).

According to DelveInsight Business Research LLP (2018), current epidemiological trends suggest there are probably as many as 250 to 300 documented cases of NPC in the United States, but the number may be much higher due to late diagnosis of the disorder. The prevalence of NPC in European countries such as France, the United Kingdom, and Germany is approximately 1 in 120,000 to 1 in 150,000 living births, primarily based on diagnostic data. It is also interesting to note that only an estimated 30 to 40 patients with a diagnosis of NPC have been identified in the country of Japan, and 25 to 30 of these are taking treatment. This demonstrates that even though the cases in Japan are remarkably low, treatment rate is much higher than in other countries (DelveInsight Business Research LLP, 2018).

Patients with NPC are often described as having a neurovisceral disorder. The visceral disorders are manifested in liver, spleen, and lung disorders. The neurologic disorders consist of dysphagia, dysarthria, cerebellar ataxia, and dementia. Most patients also exhibit vertical supranuclear gaze palsy, which is difficulty achieving upward and or downward eye movement, as well as cataplexy seizures and dystonia (Solomon, Winkelman, Zee, Gray & Büttner-Ennever, 2005). Of significance is the fact that in NPC, age plays an important role in distinguishing neurological and visceral symptoms. NPC is a fatal disease, with the majority of children dying before the age of 10. However, later onset of symptoms of the disease can lead to longer life spans, but it is unusual for individuals with NPC to surpass the fourth decade of life.

Clinical Presentation

Dysphagia is present in most patients with NPC. It can range from intermittent swallowing difficulties to complete loss of swallowing function, thus requiring alternative feeding method such as a nasogastric tube or gastrostomy. Epidemiological reports suggest that bronchopneumonia is a major cause of mortality in NPC (Walterfang et al., 2012). It is well established that dysphagia resulting from neurological disorders such as strokes and some dementias are primarily due to impairments in the oral and pharyngeal phases of the swallow and not so much from the esophageal phase. In NPC, the dysphagia appears to result from the bulbar motor dysfunction, dystonia, and the reduced sensation (Walterfang et al., 2012). Thus, it is not surprising that most patients with NPC exhibit pharyngeal dysphagia. Impairments of the pharyngeal swallowing function appear to occur later than oral-phase impairment in the course of NPC. More severe pharyngeal-phase involvement has been associated with penetration and aspiration in patients with severe overall neurological impairment (Fecarotta et al., 2011). Many patients at some point in the disease course exhibit dysphagia ranging in severity from occasional swallowing difficulties to complete loss of swallowing function, necessitating placement of nasogastric or gastrostomy feeding tubes. Patients with more severe neurological involvement generally have more severe dysphagia, and worsening neurological involvement correlates with a higher risk of aspirating food or fluid.

Prevalence of Dysphagia in NPC

According to reports from a database of 14,664 patients with neurodegenerative diseases as well as NPC, 4,065 (28%) had dysphagia. Of this number, 55% with NPC were reported to have some form of dysphagia. In fact, dysphagia in some form is prevalent in NPC and is a frequent cause of morbidity and disability (Wraith et al., 2009). Although reports differ, per reports by Walterfang et al. (2012), dysphagia in NPC ranks the second highest (55%) compared to other neurodegenerative diseases. It may occur early in the course of the disease or later, starting with simple choking or coughing, especially with liquids.

Management of Dysphagia

Management of NPC has traditionally been with symptomatic treatments that alleviate aspects of the disease and improve quality of life. Until recently, there was no disease-modifying treatment for NPC.

Speech therapy has been utilized to minimize the risk of aspiration and physical therapy has been utilized for gait disturbances; both can be effective in reducing the risks associated with the clinical manifestations of NPC. These supportive measures prolong the lives of patients by preventing hospitalizations from falls or aspirations, the latter often leading to pneumonia and death. Supportive therapies tend to be variably effective for the alleviation of clinical manifestations of NPC. Many patients have experienced relatively improved quality of life secondary to some supportive therapy.

Deficits in swallowing typically occur late in the disease course in all patients. Assessment can be performed according to the standard protocol implemented by the speech-language pathologist. Usually, a clinical swallow assessment also known as the Bedside Swallow Evaluation is carried out initially, followed by a radiographic imaging/video fluoroscopic/modified barium swallow performed using simple food textures and various liquid viscosities (thin, thickened liquids, puree, soft textures, and solids).

Current treatment of dysphagia in NPC is directed toward the specific symptoms apparent in each individual. Dysphagia should be monitored and evaluated regularly for the risk of aspiration. Standard clinical and instrumental evaluation of the swallowing difficulties are typically performed by the speech-language pathologist. The treatment protocol is based on the nature of the swallowing problem. Since most patients with NPC initially present with poor control of liquids, the viscosity of the liquids may be manipulated to suit the patient as determined through the modified barium swallow studies. Solid foods may also be modified to softer textures as well based on the patient's swallowing ability. Eventually, a gastronomy tube may be required to meet adequate caloric needs. With this procedure, a thin tube is placed into the stomach via a small incision in the abdomen, allowing for the direct intake of food or medicine.

Managing and treating dysphagia in NPC serves only to lessen the burden of the disease but in no way changes its underlying course. While there is no known cure for the disease, there has been some positive strides made with a miglustat, also known as N-butyldeoxynojirimycin. Miglustat is a drug recently approved for the treatment of NPC in adults, adolescents, and children. It was approved in many European countries in 2009, in Canada in 2010, and in Japan in 2012, but not in the United States where the Food and Drug Administration (FDA) declined to approve it, requesting more data. However, to date, there are some encouraging results from a number of NPC patients 12 years of age and older. After a year of treatment with miglustat, there was significant improvement. Individuals showed improvement in the neurological disorders associated with NPC. Walterfang et al. (2012) provided a systematic report of the progress that has been made in several clinical trials worldwide detailing the use of miglustat (Table 2–1).

Summary

Niemann-Pick disease type C is a rare and fatal neurovisceral lipid-storage disease that affects both children and adults. To date, the data are sparse in terms of the incidence and prevalence. Management of NPC has historically been with symptomatic treatments to alleviate certain aspects of the disease and mostly to improve quality of life. Among the many and varied sequelae of disorders secondary to this disease, dysphagia is one of the more prevalent ones and is categorized as one of the neurological presentations of the disorder. While there is no cure for NPC, one of the most promising drugs used to treat the disease is miglustat. This has been approved in some European countries, Canada,

Table 2–1. Summary of Randomized and Nonrandomized Studies with Information on the Effects of Miglustat on Dysphagia

Trial ID [reference]	Design	Treatment	Patients	Swallowing Function	Key Findings
OGT-918-007	12-month, randomized, controlled, Phase II study comparing miglustat with standard (symptomatic) therapy	Main study: miglustat 200 mg t.i.d. ($n=20$) vs. standard care ($n=9$) Substudy: miglustat 200 mg t.i.d. adjusted for BSA ($n=12$)	Main study: male and female adults and juveniles (aged ≥ 12 years) Substudy: male and female children aged 4–11 years	Ability to swallow different foods (5 mL of water, 1 teaspoon of puree, 1 teaspoon of soft lumps, or a third of a cookie) Assessed at 6 and 12 months or withdrawal/follow-up	Improved ability to swallow water in 6 patients (30%), puree in 3 patients (15%), soft lumps in 3 patients (15%), and a third of a cookie in 7 patients (35%) after 12 months of miglustat therapy More than 80% of children had normal swallowing at baseline

continues

Table 2-1. *continued*

Trial ID [reference]	Design	Treatment	Patients	Swallowing Function	Key Findings
OGT-918-007 ext (a)	Prospective, noncontrolled, 12-month extension to OGT-918-007	Miglustat 200 mg t.i.d.	Male and female adults and juveniles (aged ≥12 years) who received miglustat (n=17) or standard care (n=8) for 12 months	Swallowing assessment (as above) at 12 and 24 months and last visit	Swallowing improved/stable (vs. baseline) in 86% of patients completing 12 months on miglustat, and 79–93% of those completing 24 months on miglustat
OGT-918-007 ext (b)	Prospective, non-controlled, 12-month extension to OGT-918-007 substudy	Miglustat 200 mg t.i.d. adjusted for BSA	Male and female children aged 4–11 years who underwent 12 months of miglustat therapy (n=10)	Swallowing assessment (as above) at 12 and 24 months and last visit	Nine patients (90%) had normal swallowing function at both baseline and 24 months

30

Table 2–1. *continued*

Trial ID [reference]	Design	Treatment	Patients	Swallowing Function	Key Findings
NP-C Retrospective Stage 1 Survey	Retrospective, multicenter, observational, cohort study	Adults ≥18 years (*n* = 14): miglustat 200 mg t.i.d. Juveniles 12–17 years (*n* = 13): miglustat 200 mg t.i.d. Pediatrics ≤12 years (*n* = 34): miglustat adjusted for BSA	Patients previously or currently treated with miglustat in clinical practice settings	Dysphagia subscale of NPC disability scale	Continuous deterioration prior to initiation of miglustat therapy Similar proportions of patients in each swallowing disability category at treatment start and last post-treatment assessment (stabilization)
Spanish/ Portuguese Pediatric Cohort Study	Multicenter, observational chart review	Miglustat 200 mg t.i.d. adjusted for BSA in symptomatic patients (*n* = 16) Symptomatic therapy in 1 asymptomatic patient	Male and female pediatric patients treated in Spain and Portugal	Dysphagia subscale of a modified NPC disability scale	Stable neurological manifestations (including swallowing) in juvenile-onset patients Smaller therapeutic benefits in younger-onset patients with greater disease severity at baseline

continues

31

Table 2–1. *continued*

Trial ID [reference]	Design	Treatment	Patients	Swallowing Function	Key Findings
Italian Case Series	Longitudinal case series of Italian patients	Miglustat 250–300 mg/mq/day in three divided doses for up to 4 years	Male and female patients treated for ≥3 years, with swallowing function assessed by VFSS ($n=4$)	VFSS	Improved swallowing in patients with dysphagia/aspiration at baseline ($n=3$) No deterioration in the patient with normal swallowing at baseline
Taiwanese Data	Longitudinal case reports	Miglustat 200 mg t.i.d. adjusted for BSA for 1 year	Young male patients, 1 with severe swallowing impairment and 1 with impaired language/speech who underwent serial VFSS	VFSS	Patient 1: substantially improved swallowing function after 6 months Patient 2: normal swallowing before and throughout therapy

Note: BSA = body surface area; *VFSS* = videofluoroscopic studies.
Source: As reported in Walterfang et al., 2012.

and Japan, but not yet in the United States. Much is still unclear about the neuropathology of NPC. Additional data from studies are ongoing in the efforts to find a cure for NPC.

References

Crocker, A. C. (1961). The cerebral defect in Tay-Sachs disease and Niemann-Pick disease. *Journal of Neurochemistry, 7*(1), 69–80.

Davidson, C. D., & Walkley, S. U. (2010). Niemann-Pick type C disease—Pathophysiology and future perspectives for treatment. *U.S. Neurology, 8*, 88–94.

DelveInsight Business Research LLP. (2018). Niemann-Pick disease—type C—Epidemiology trends, *Global Information, Inc.* Retrieved from https://www.giiresearch.com/report/del650463-niemann-pick -disease-type-c-npc-market-insights.html

Fecarotta, S., Amitrano, M., Romano, A., Della Casa, R., Bruschini, D., Astarita, L., . . . Andria, G. (2011). The videofluoroscopic swallowing study shows a sustained improvement of dysphagia in children with Niemann–Pick disease type C after therapy with miglustat. *American Journal of Medical Genetics Part A, 155*(3), 540–547.

Fink, J. K. (2004). Niemann-Pick disease. In L. R. Squire (Ed.), *Encyclopedia of Neuroscience* (pp. 1141–1144). Cambridge, MA: Academic Press.

Niemann-Pick disease. (2019). *Genetic and Rare Disease Information Center (GARD)*. Retrieved from https://rarediseases.info.nih.gov /diseases/13334/niemann-pick-disease

Public Health England. (2015, September 18). *Improving outcomes for babies with genetic disorders.* Retrieved from https://phescreening .blog.gov.uk/2015/09/18/improving-outcomes-for-babies-with -genetic-disorders/

Sevin, M., Lesca, G., Baumann, N., Millat, G., Lyon-Caen, O., Vanier, M. T., & Sedel, F. (2007). The adult form of Niemann-Pick disease type C. *Brain, 130*(Pt. 1), 120–133.

Solomon, D., Winkelman, A. C., Zee, D. S., Gray, L., & Büttner-Ennever, J. E. A. N. (2005). Niemann-Pick type C disease in two affected sisters: Ocular motor recordings and brain-stem neuropathology. *Annals of the New York Academy of Sciences, 1039*(1), 436–445.

Trendelenburg, G., Vanier, M. T., Maza, S., Millat, G., Bohner, G., Munz, D. L., & Zschenderlein, R. (2006). Niemann-Pick type C disease in a 68-year-old patient. *Journal of Neurology, Neurosurgery, & Psychiatry, 77*(8), 997–998.

Vanier, M. T. (2010). Niemann-Pick disease type C. *Orphanet Journal of Rare Diseases, 5*(1), 16.

Walterfang, M., Chien, Y. H., Imrie, J., Rushton, D., Schubiger, D., & Patterson, M. C. (2012). Dysphagia as a risk factor for mortality in Niemann-Pick disease type C: Systematic literature review and evidence from studies with miglustat. *Orphanet Journal of Rare Diseases, 7*(1), 76.

Wraith, J. E., Guffon, N., Rohrbach, M., Hwu, W. L., Korenke, G. C., Bembi, B., . . . Sedel, F. (2009). Natural history of Niemann-Pick disease type C in a multicentre observational retrospective cohort study. *Molecular Genetics and Metabolism, 98*(3), 250–254.

3

Stuve-Wiedemann Syndrome

KEY WORDS: Stuve-Wiedemann syndrome, hypotonia, hyperthermia, scoliosis, hypokinesia, camptodactyly, consanguineous

Definition

Stuve-Wiedemann syndrome (SWS) is a rare, severe, autosomal recessive condition characterized by bone abnormalities and dysfunction of the autonomic nervous system, resulting in **hypotonia**, respiratory distress/apneic spells, and episodes of dangerously high body temperatures (**hyperthermia**; Bonthuis, Morava, Booij, & Driessen, 2009). Many infants with SWS do not survive because of difficulty regulating breathing and body temperature; however, some individuals with SWS survive into adolescence and beyond. Moreover, the dysfunction of the autonomic nervous system typically leads to feeding and swallowing difficulties that accompany SWS. Even though in many cases the problems with respiration and swallowing usually get better in those children who survive, they continue to have difficulty regulating body temperature. Rare survivors of SWS develop progressive scoliosis, spontaneous fractures, bowing of the lower limbs with prominent joints, absent corneal and patellar reflexes, and smooth tongue.

History

Stüve and Wiedemann (1971) described the first cases of SWS. Two sisters and a cousin presented with congenital bowing of the tibia and femur, abnormally positioned feet, and **camptodactyly** (permanently bent fingers). They both suffered respiratory distress. One of the siblings exhibited feeding problems as well as hyperthermia, but all died within the neonatal period. An autosomal recessive pattern of inheritance was evident since there was the recurrent pattern of the disorder in both siblings as well as a first cousin (Bertola, Honjo, & Baratela, 2016). Several years later, the eponym Stuve-Wiedemann syndrome was recognized.

Admittedly, the identification of SWS as a disorder took many years. This was most likely due to the overlapping characteristics between SWS and a subtype of Schwartz-Jampel syndrome (SJS). Both disorders have presentations of prenatal onset of **hypokinesia**, congenital contractures, feeding difficulties, early lethality, and a distinct radiological pattern of congenital bowing of the long bones, myotonia, and other skeletal abnormalities (Bertola et al., 2016). This overlap in the two disorders based on their clinical and radiologic presentations led researchers and geneticists to conclude that SJS type 2 and SWS were actually a single disorder (Superti-Furga et al.,1998); thus, the term Schwartz-Jampel syndrome has given way to the more commonly used Stuve-Wiedemann syndrome.

Etiology

SWS is an inherited autosomal recessive trait caused by a change (mutation) in the leukemia inhibitory factor receptor (LIFR) gene. Most genetic diseases are determined by the status of the two copies of a gene, one received from the father and one from the mother. Recessive genetic disorders occur when an individual inherits two copies of an abnormal gene for the same trait, one from each parent. Consanguineous parents have a higher chance than unrelated parents to both carry the same abnormal gene, which increases the risk to have children with a recessive genetic disorder (NORD, 2018).

Most of the SWS cases reported are associated with a mutation in the LIFR gene (Mikelonis, Jorcyk, Tawara, & Oxford, 2014). LIFR acts as a receptor for a molecule known as leukemia inhibitory factor (LIF). LIFR controls several cellular processes such as growth and division (proliferation), maturation (differentiation), and survival. LIFR is important in blocking (inhibiting) growth of blood cancer (leukemia) cells. This signaling is also involved in the formation of bone and the development of nerve cells. It is also involved in the normal development and functioning of the autonomic nervous system, which controls involuntary body processes such as the regulation of breathing rate, body temperature, and swallowing (Dagoneau et al., 2004).

Even in the rare disorder of SWS there is genetic variability. For example, not all patients with SWS have an identified LIFR mutation (Al Kaissi, Rumpler, Csepan, Grill, & Klaushofer, 2008). In these cases, it appears that the gene(s) responsible for the phenotypic presentation of SWS have not been identified (Mikelonis et al., 2014).

Epidemiology

While SWS has a low prevalence of less than 1 in 1 million, but it is relatively common in the United Arab Emirates with an incidence of 1 in 20,000 births. This frequency may be because parents are often closely related (**consanguineous**). The disease occurs in both males and females equally. In spite of its rarity, SWS has been described in multiple ethnic groups, including individuals from European countries (Dagoneau et al., 2004; Wiedemann & Stüve, 1996), Africa (Cormier-Daire et al., 1998), North and South America (Chen, Cotter, Cohen, & Lachman, 2001), and the Middle East (Dagoneau et al., 2004).

Clinical Presentation

The main distinguishing features of SWS are the skeletal manifestations including osteopenia, dwarfism, and bowing of the long bones. Most affected children present with bowing limbs early at the neonatal period (Figure 3–1). Facial features usually include short palpebral fissures and pursing of the mouth, especially on stimulation. Additional features include camptodactyly, figure contractures, and signs and symptoms of dysautonomia. Table 3–1 presents the common characteristics of SWS. Most individuals diagnosed with SWS do not survive beyond 10 months. This failure to survive is mostly due to respiratory distress, feeding and swallowing difficulties, as well as hyperthermic episodes (Wiedmann & Stüve, 1996). However, patients that do survive do so because of improved respiratory and swallowing.

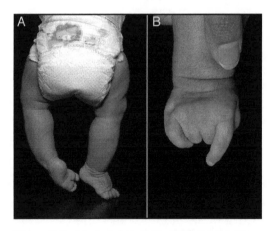

Figure 3–1. Limb deformity in SWS. *Source*: From "Stuve-Wiedemann syndrome with a novel mutation case," by M. Knipe, R. Stanbury, S. Unger, and M. Chakraborty, 2015, *British Medical Journal Case Report, 30*. doi:10.1136/bcr-2015-212032

Table 3–1. Diagnostic Characteristics of SWS

Organ System	Neonate	Childhood
Embryonic	Oligohydramnios intrauterine growth restriction, low birth weight	Growth retardation
Skeletal	Micromelia, bowing of long bones, camptodactyly, scoliosis, facial anomalies	Bowing of long bones, camptodactyly, scoliosis, facial anomalies
Muscular	Hypotonia, contractures	
Pulmonary	Respiratory distress, pulmonary hypoplasia	Improvement of respiratory distress
Cardiovascular	Pulmonary hypertension	
Gastrointestinal	Dysphagia: feeding problems	Dysphagia

Clinical Presentation of Dysphagia in SWS

The course of SWS in the neonatal period and throughout infancy for those who survive is characterized by episodes of hyperthermia as well as feeding and swallowing difficulties. The swallowing problems often lead to aspiration pneumonia and in many cases death. It is proposed that the swallowing difficulties manifested in patients with SWS may be directly related to an impaired autonomic system. Apparently, the pharyngoesophageal dyskinesia in SWS secondary to dysautonomia occurs because of an abnormal control of the anterior rami of cervical roots at the level of C1–C5 (Corona-Rivera et al., 2009).

Corona-Rivera et al. (2009) observed oropharyngeal dysphagia in one SWS patient. This patient repeated episodes of aspiration pneumonia.

SWS is diagnosed based on clinical as well as radiologic findings after birth. Although prenatal ultrasounds can be helpful in diagnosing the disorder, the main ultrasound findings in SWS must be differentiated from other diseases with bent bone dysplasias (Begam et al., 2011). Nevertheless, most of the identified cases of SWS have had a positive family history; therefore, history is critical in making the diagnosis.

Radiological findings are critical for a positive diagnosis of SWS. These images show the congenital contractures, bowed long bones, decreased bone density, and other abnormal patterns. The elbow and knee joints appear deformed, fingers and feet are malpositioned, and **scoliosis** is present (Bertola et al., 2016). The main distinguishing features of SWS are the skeletal manifestations including osteopenia, dwarfism, and bowing of the long bones.

Management of Dysphagia

Unfortunately, there is no specific treatment available for SWS. Consequently, treatment involves managing the symptoms with which each patient presents. In terms of dysphagia, the priority is to prevent aspiration pneumonia, which is the main cause of death in the first few months of life. Many of the affected infants require nasogastric tube feedings or gastrostomy at some point in infancy and well into childhood (Akawi, Ali, & Al-Gazali, 2012). The speech-language pathologist plays a critical role in assessing the nature of the swallowing problem, particularly as the surviving child gets older. As the affected surviving child gets older, swallowing tends to become more normal. Even in such cases, the child may show intermittent swallowing deficits. One of the manifestations in dysautonomia is decreased sensation and smooth tongue; consequently, it is not surprising that tongue injury is a frequent occurrence. This can be managed by the use of a device to cover the teeth until the child is old enough to understand how to avoid this behavior.

As previously noted, patients with SWS who survive the first year of life tend to improve in their ability to swallow as well as to regulate their breathing. This is an exceptional improvement as swallowing difficulties, as well as respiratory and hyperthermic episodes, are the most frequent causes of early deaths in SWS.

Summary

SWS is a rare, autosomal recessive, inherited disease of a mutated LIFR with manifestations of bent bone dysplasia and dysautonomia. These symptoms of SWS result from a lack of LIFR signaling, mechanisms of which are still largely unclear. There is no treatment available for SWS; however, symptoms of the disease are the focus of treatment. Prognosis of SWS continues to be poor. Further research is needed to provide a better understanding of the disease and to identify appropriate treatment protocols.

References

Akawi, N. A., Ali, B. R., & Al-Gazali, L. (2012). Stüve-Wiedemann syndrome and related bent bone dysplasias. *Clinical Genetics, 82*(1), 12–21.

Al Kaissi, A., Rumpler, M., Csepan, R., Grill, F., & Klaushofer, K. (2008). Congenital contractures and distinctive phenotypic features consistent with Stüve-Wiedmann syndrome in a male infant. *Cases Journal, 1*(1), 121.

Begam, M. A., Alsafi, W., Bekdache, G. N., Chedid, F., Al-Gazali, L., & Mirghani, H. M. (2011). Stüve-Wiedemann syndrome: A skeletal dysplasia characterized by bowed long bones. *Ultrasound in Obstetrics & Gynecology, 38*(5), 553–558.

Bertola, D. R., Honjo, R. S., & Baratela, W. A. (2016). Stüve-Wiedemann syndrome: Update on clinical and genetic aspects. *Molecular Syndromology, 7*(1), 12–18.

Bonthuis, D., Morava, E., Booij, L. H., & Driessen, J. J. (2009). Stüve Wiedemann syndrome and related syndromes: Case report and possible anesthetic complications. *Pediatric Anesthesia, 19*(3), 212–217.

Chen, E., Cotter, P. D., Cohen, R. A., & Lachman, R. S. (2001). Characterization of a long-term survivor with Stüve-Wiedemann syndrome and mosaicism of a supernumerary marker chromosome. *American Journal of Medical Genetics, 101*(3), 240–245.

Cormier-Daire, V., Superti-Furga, A., Munnich, A., Lyonnet, S., Rustin, P., Delezoide, A. L., . . . Le Merrer, M. (1998). Clinical homogeneity of the Stüve-Wiedemann syndrome and overlap with the Schwartz-Jampel syndrome type 2. *American Journal of Medical Genetics, 78*(2), 146–149.

Corona-Rivera, J. R., Cormier-Daire, V., Dagoneau, N., Coello-Ramírez, P., López-Marure, E., Romo-Huerta, C. O., . . . Estrada-Solorio, M. I. (2009). Abnormal oral-pharyngeal swallowing as cause of morbidity and early death in Stüve-Wiedemann syndrome. *European Journal of Medical Genetics, 52*(4), 242–246.

Dagoneau, N., Scheffer, D., Huber, C., Al-Gazali, L. I., Di Rocco, M., Godard, A., . . . Cormier-Daire, V. (2004). Null leukemia inhibitory factor receptor (LIFR) mutations in Stüve-Wiedemann/Schwartz-Jampel type 2 syndrome. *The American Journal of Human Genetics, 74*(2), 298–305.

Knipe, M., Stanbury, R., Unger, S., & Chakraborty, M. (2015). Stuve-Wiedemann syndrome with a novel mutation case. *BMJ Case Rep, 30.* doi:10.1136/bcr-2015-212032

Mikelonis, D., Jorcyk, C. L., Tawara, K., & Oxford, J. T. (2014). Stüve-Wiedemann syndrome: LIFR and associated cytokines in clinical course and etiology. *Orphanet Journal of Rare Diseases, 9*(1), 34.

NORD. (2018). *Stuve-Wiedemann syndrome. Genetic and rare diseases information center.* Retrieved February 1, 2018, from https://rerediseases .info.nih.gov/diseases/5045/stuve-wiedemann-syndrome

Stüve, A., & Wiedemann, H. R. (1971). Congenital bowing of the long bones in two sisters. *Lancet, 298*(7722), 495.

Superti-Furga, A., Tenconi, R., Clementi, M., Eich, G., Steinmann, B., Boltshauser, E., & Giedion, A. (1998). Schwartz-Jampel syndrome type 2 and Stüve-Wiedemann syndrome: A case for "Lumping." *American Journal of Medical Genetics, 78*(2), 150–154.

Wiedemann, H. R., & Stüve, A. (1996). Stüve-Wiedemann syndrome: Update and historical footnote. *American Journal of Medical Genetics, 63*(1), 12–16.

4

Congenital Esophageal Stenosis

KEY WORDS: congenital esophageal stenosis, esophageal atresia, achalasia, esophagram

Definition

Congenital esophageal stenosis (CES) is a rare developmental disorder that causes significant dysphagia. It is described as a failure of complete separation of the respiratory tract from the primitive gut in early fetal development. CES is often associated with esophageal atresia. In esophageal atresia, the esophagus fails to connect normally to the stomach; instead, it ends in a blind-ended pouch. Failure of the separation process of the trachea and the esophagus can result in three types of CES: (1) tracheobronchial remnants (TBR) in the esophageal wall—this type tends to involve the lower third of the esophagus; (2) fibromuscular stenosis (FMS)/hypertrophy of the muscle and submucosal layers; and (3) membranous diaphragm or membranous stenosis (MD/MS). Both FMS and MD/MS tend to occur in the middle third of the esophagus.

History

Frey and Duschli reported the earliest case of CES in 1936. They described the case of a 19-year-old girl whose death was attributed to the diagnosis of achalasia and who was found to have cartilage in the cardia. The classification of CES has been confusing mainly because it is a rare condition. To date, various classifications of CES have been proposed. Nihoul-Fekete (1987) defined CES and categorized the cases based on three entities. This categorization continues to be broadly accepted. According to Nihoul-Fekete, CES is either due to fibromuscular thickening, tracheobronchial remnants (TBR), or membranous web. Fibromuscular thickening is found to be the most frequent of these entities, followed by TBR and membranous web. TBR are often encircling cartilaginous rings within the wall of the esophagus.

Etiology

Congenital esophageal stenosis (CES) results from an incomplete separation of the respiratory tract from the primitive foregut at the 25th day of life. Embryologically, the primitive gut tube develops around weeks 3 to 4. In this process, craniocaudal and lateral folding of the embryo occurs (Figure 4–1). At this stage of development, the tube is divided into three sections: the foregut, the midgut, and the hindgut. The esophagus, stomach, liver, gallbladder and bile ducts, pancreas, and the duodenum will arise from the foregut. During this period, lateral grooves on the sides of the foregut invaginate and eventually fuse, creating a septum or common wall, thus separating the trachea from the esophagus. Any error in this separation process will result in some esophageal abnormality such as stenosis, atresia, or a fistula.

While CES is a rare clinical condition, other similar conditions such as **esophageal atresia** (see Chapter 14) and esophageal fistula also give rise to persistent and profound dysphagia.

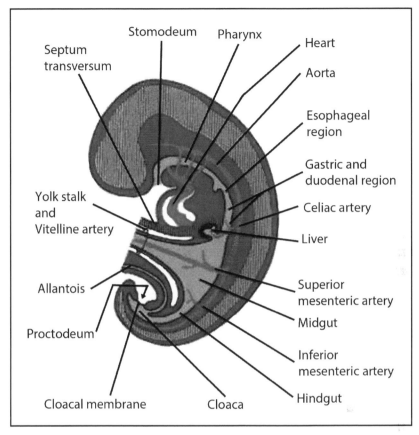

Figure 4–1. Embryonic primordial gut at 4 weeks. *Source*: From *The developing human* (7th ed.), by K. L. Moore and T. V. N. Persaud, 2003, Philadelphia, PA: Elsevier, Inc.

For example, in an extensive longitudinal study conducted by Michaud et al. (2013), over an 18-year period, 61 patients had CES and 29 of these had esophageal atresia associated with the CES. Forty of the 61 children with CES had esophageal atresia. All three types of CES—tracheobronchial remnants (TBR), fibromuscular stenosis (FMS), and membrane stenosis (MS)—were seen across all patients.

CES is a rare disorder with currently about 500 reported cases in the published literature (Ramesh, Ramanujam, & Jayaram, 2017). Each type of CES differs based on specific location in the

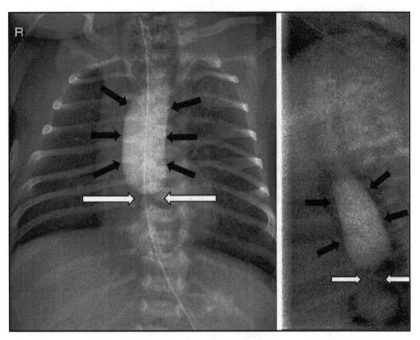

Figure 4–2. Stenosis of the distal esophagus. *Source*: From "An unusual presentation of congenital esophageal stenosis due to tracheobronchial remnants in a newborn prenatally diagnosed with duodenal atresia," by C. Mai, L. Breysem, G. De Hertogh, D. Van Raemdonck, and M. H. Smet, 2015, *Journal of the Belgian Society of Radiology, 99*(2), 43–46. doi:http://doi.org/10.5334/jbr-btr.881.

esophagus. CES of the TBR and FMS types tends to involve a length of the esophageal wall, whereas CES of the MS type involves the mucosal folds and not the muscular layer (Figure 4–2).

As the name suggests, CES is a condition that is present at birth, and most research suggest that the uterine environment most likely causes it. So far, there are no reports to substantiate it as a genetically linked disorder. Nevertheless, it is of interest to note that presently, two cases with a familial link have been reported in the literature. Harrison and Katon (1992) reported the case of a 35-year-old male with multiple esophageal rings and severe dysphagia whose father suffered similar symptoms. In a similar report, Rangel and Lizarzabel (1998) reported the case of a 47-year-old female from Venezuela with a history of esophageal rings that caused her to have dysphagia for solids. Her sibling reportedly suffered from a similar condition. While these two cases do not support a claim for CES as an inherited disorder, it certainly does open the door for more probing.

Epidemiology

The incidence of CES is reportedly 1 per 25,000 to 50,000 live births. It is commonly caused by congenital malformation, gastroesophageal reflux, and **achalasia** (Singh, Ansari, Gupta, Sharma, & Goyal, 2014). Even though CES occurs in both males and females, there is a slight male predominance. In a review of 132 cases, Kim, Kim, Jung, Lee, and Park (2017) reported a male predominance with a ratio of 70:62 boys to girls However, there does not appear to be a substantiated medical reason for this predominance. While CES is a rare clinical condition, other similar conditions such as esophageal atresia and esophageal fistula also give rise to the persistent and profound dysphagia present. For example, in an extensive longitudinal study conducted by Michaud et al. (2013), over an 18-year period, 61 patients had CES and 29 of these had esophageal atresia associated with the CES.

The rarity of CES has been well documented, but the true incidence is still relatively unknown (Terui, Saito, Mitsunaga, Nakata, & Yoshida, 2015). There are reports that suggest less rarity of CES when it presents with esophageal atresia (EA) and/or tracheoesophageal fistula (TEF). In their review of published CES cases, Terui et al. (2015) reported a higher incidence rate (25%) of EA and/or TEF in patients with CES (Table 4–1).

Most cases of CES are reported in children. It is a challenge to substantiate whether the adult cases are truly congenital. As previously reported in Chapter 1 of this text, esophageal webs are systemic to the diagnosis of Plummer-Vinson syndrome. Terui et al. (2015) cited the largest cases of adult CES in which 62% of the cases with upper esophageal webs also had anemia. CES is usually diagnosed in infants soon after birth and certainly within

Table 4–1. Incidence Rate of Esophageal Atresia and/or Tracheoesophageal Fistula Among Patients with Congenital Esophageal Stenosis

Reference	Cases	Incidence Rate	EA	EA + TEF	TEF
Bluestone et al. (1969)	0/24	0.0%	0	0	0
Nishina et al. (1981)	4/81	4.9%	0	3	1
Dominguez et al. (1985)	5/34	14.7%	0	5	0
Nihoul-Fékété et al. (1987)	2/20	10.0%	0	1	1
Yeung et al. (1992)	6/8	75.0%	1	4	1
Vasudevan et al. (2002)	4/6	66.7%	1	2	1
Takamizawa et al. (2002)	13/36	36.1%	0	13	0
Amae et al. (2003)	4/14	28.6%	0	4	0
Romeo et al. (2011)	15/47	31.9%	0	15	0
Michaud et al. (2013)	29/61	47.5%	0	29	0
Total	82/331	24.8%	2 (2.4%)	76 (92.7%)	4 (4.9%)

months. However, in adults, it tends to be underrecognized. This may be related to the severity of the signs and symptoms, as some individuals may be able to tolerate mild dysphagia without reporting it. Younes and Johnson (1999) studied 10 patients over a 7-year period, eight males and two females ranging in age from 21 to 75 years. All of the patients had segmental esophageal stenosis due to multiple submucosal rings. All of the patients reported some form of dysphagia over 10 to 40 years. Younes and Johnson suggested that in adults, CES may be an underrecognized cause of dysphagia and hence not diagnosed earlier.

Clinical Presentation

CES is frequently diagnosed in young children. Many reports have indicated that typical symptoms appear during the period when the infant is transitioning from breastmilk or formula to solid foods. For the most part, many patients feed well at birth, and then dysphagic symptoms appear insidiously into adulthood.

Kim, Kim, Jung, Lee, and Park (2017) studied 31 patients with CES. The age at the first dysphagia symptom presentation ranged from 1 day to 10 years, and the age at diagnosis ranged from 8 days to 12 years. These authors found that the most common symptom in all of their patients was vomiting, followed by food or foreign body impaction as well as frequent respiratory infection (Table 4–2).

Dysphagia is the main clinical symptom in the diagnosis CES. Of the three types of CES previously discussed—TBR, FMS and MS—TBR, the most common type, affects the lower third of the esophagus, while the other two types affect the region of the middle third of the esophagus. CES of the TBR type tends to cause vomiting; whereas, the other two types cause more respiratory problems (Serrao, Santos, Gaivao, Tavares, & Ferreira, 2010).

The diagnosis of CES is usually difficult to make on clinical grounds only. The rarity of the disease and the relative lack of awareness of this disorder by many physicians result in late diagnosis. Three key elements to a diagnosis of CES are (1) a high

Table 4–2. Common Clinical Characteristics of Patients with Congenital Esophageal Stenosis

Gender	Age at Diagnosis (Year & Months)	Associated Anomalies	Symptoms	Degree of Stenosis	Type of Stenosis
Female	6.6	None	Vomiting, dysphagia, respiratory infection	Severe	TBR
Male	4.0	None	Vomiting, dysphagia, respiratory infection	Severe	TBR
Male	8.0	Club foot	Vomiting, respiratory infection	Severe	TBR
Female	2.11	Cardiac	Vomiting, foreign body impaction	Severe	TBR
Female	2.9	None	Vomiting	Severe	TBR
Male	2.10	Down syndrome, cardiac	Vomiting	Severe	TBR
Female	2.9	None	Vomiting	Severe	TBR
Male	5.1	None	Vomiting	Severe	TBR
Female	1.5	None	Vomiting, food impaction	Moderate	TBR

Table 4–2. *continued*

Gender	Age at Diagnosis (Year & Months)	Associated Anomalies	Symptoms	Degree of Stenosis	Type of Stenosis
Male	10 months	None	Vomiting, food impaction	Severe	TBR
Female	9.11	Down syndrome	Vomiting	Moderate	TBR
Male	6.2	Imperforate anus	Vomiting	Moderate	TBR
Male	7.1	None	Vomiting	Moderate	TBR
Female	1.2	None	Vomiting	Moderate	TBR
Male	9 months	None	Vomiting, respiratory infection, dysphagia	Moderate	FMH
Female	2.3	None	Vomiting	Severe	TBR
Female	1.7	None	Vomiting	Moderate	TBR
Male	1.2	None	Vomiting	Moderate	TBR
Male	8.6	Club-foot	Vomiting	Severe	TBR

continues

Table 4–2. *continued*

Gender	Age at Diagnosis (Year & Months)	Associated Anomalies	Symptoms	Degree of Stenosis	Type of Stenosis
Male	12.5	Annular pancreas with duodenal atresia	Dysphagia	Moderate	TBR
Female	1.9	None	Vomiting	Severe	TBR
Female	2.0	Imperforate anus	Vomiting	Moderate	TBR
Female	8 months	Esophageal-atresia with tracheo-esophageal fistula	Vomiting, respiratory Infection, dysphagia	Severe	TBR
Male	13 days	Esophageal-atresia with tracheo-esophageal fistula	Vomiting	Severe	TBR
Male	3.0	Esophageal-atresia with tracheo-esophageal fistula	Vomiting	Severe	TBR
Female	7 months	Esophageal-atresia with tracheo-esophageal fistula, imperforate anus, annular pancreas with duodenal atresia	Vomiting, food impaction	Moderate	FMH

Table 4–2. *continued*

Gender	Age at Diagnosis (Year & Months)	Associated Anomalies	Symptoms	Degree of Stenosis	Type of Stenosis
Female	14 days	Esophageal-atresia with tracheo-esophageal fistula, cardiac anomaly	Vomiting	Moderate	TBR
Male	11 days	Esophageal-atresia with tracheoesophageal fistula	Vomiting, food impaction	Severe	FMH
Male	20 days	Esophageal-atresia with tracheo-esophageal fistula	Vomiting, food impaction, dysphagia	Severe	TBR
Female	2.7	Esophageal-atresia with tracheoesophageal fistula	Vomiting, dysphagia	Proximal: moderate; Distal: severe	TBR
Male	8 days	Esophageal-atresia with tracheo-esophageal fistula	Vomiting, food impaction	Moderate	TBR

Legend: Tracheobronchial remnants (TBR) and fibromuscular hypertrophy (FMH).

Source: Adapted from information in "Clinical study of congenital esophageal stenosis: Comparison according to Association of Esophageal Atresia and Tracheoesophageal Fistula," by S. H. Kim, H. Y. Kim, S. E. Jung, S. C. Lee, & K. W. Park, 2017, *Pediatric Gastroenterology, Hepatology & Nutrition, 20*(2), 79–86.

level of suspicion, (2) accurate history regarding the time of onset and the nature of the symptoms, and (3) radiological reports such as an **esophagram**. Nevertheless, a definitive diagnosis can only be rendered postoperatively in most cases (Ibrahim, Al, Malki, Hamza, & Bahnassy, 2007). According to Serrao et al. (2010), an endoscopic evaluation will not only identify the stenosis, but will rule out esophagitis and foreign bodies. With the advancement of medical technology, including endoscopic ultrasonography, magnetic resonance imaging (MRI), as well as CT-scans with contrast, there are various useful tools currently available for providing an accurate diagnosis (Serrao et al., 2010). Even though these methods of diagnosis are critical to identification of the CES, definitive diagnosis still relies on the histological tests (Ramesh et al., 2001; Zhao, Hsieh, & Hsu, 2004)

Management of Dysphagia

The management of CES depends on the pathologic type. For patients with the MD type, balloon dilatation and endoscopic incision can result in improvement. According to Serrao et al. (2010), in FMH patients, esophageal dilatation has shown improvements, but it does not always have an effect. In some studies, TBR patients experienced no benefit from dilatation. On the other hand, other studies have shown complete resolution of stenosis and symptoms after dilatation alone, even for TBR patients. Yet, other research suggested that for TBR patients, balloon dilatation might be effective. However, the main treatment for esophageal stricture is still through dilation. In this procedure, the esophagus is stretched by the use of either multiple dilators or an air-filled balloon that is passed through an endoscope. While this therapy treats the vast majority of strictures, repeated dilation may be necessary to prevent the stricture from returning. In fact, a recurring stricture is reported to occur in about 30% of people after dilation within the first year. It is a common practice for most patients to be prescribed certain medications such as Prilosec, Lansoproprazole, or Rabeprazole following the surgical procedure. But in most cases, surgery tends to be the last resort for treating esophageal stenosis. It is performed when the dilatation of the stricture fails to allow the person to swallow both liquids and solids.

Fundoplication is one type of surgical procedure for managing CES. In fundoplication, the part of the stomach that is closest to the esophagus, the *fundus,* is gathered, wrapped, and sutured around the lower esophageal area. This process of gathering and suturing is called *"plication,"* hence the term *"fundoplication."* Dysphagia is a frequent complication secondary to fundoplication. After treatment, a person can usually go back to regular routines and diets, although they may develop strictures again in the future, which may cause recurrent problems swallowing—thus the need for medications, as described previously.

Dysphagia Management

Management of dysphagia is largely dependent on the underlying cause and is directly related to the management of the stricture. In esophageal dysphagia, which often results from CES, patients frequently complain of a pressure sensation in the midchest area, especially for solid-textured foods. In children, there is often oral or pharyngeal regurgitation/spitting up, aspiration pneumonia, weight loss, or failure to thrive.

According to Easterling (2015), the speech-language pathologist (SLP) still relies on the esophagram performed by the radiologist to confirm esophageal dysphagia. However, the SLP plays a significant role in determining the appropriate texture and liquid viscosity that the individual is able to manage safely.

Summary

CES is a rare anomaly resulting from an incomplete separation of the respiratory tract from the primitive foregut at the 25th day of life. The primary clinical signs of this disorder are manifested in abnormalities of the swallowing mechanism. This type of dysphagia results largely from the stenosis of the esophagus. Diagnosis of CES is usually difficult to make on clinical grounds only. Diagnosis is typically delayed and requires a high level of suspicion of the disorder, accurate history regarding the time of onset and the nature of the symptoms, and radiological reports such as an esophagram. Nevertheless, a definitive diagnosis can only be rendered postoperatively. Treatment largely involves surgery and is contingent on the location and type of stenosis.

References

Amae, S., Nio, M., Kamiyama, T., Ishii, T., Yoshida, S., Hayashi, Y., & Ohi, R. (2003). Clinical characteristics and management of congenital esophageal stenosis: A report on 14 cases. *Journal of Pediatric Surgery, 38*(4), 565–570.

Bluestone, C. D., Kerry, R., & Sieber, W. K. (1969). Congenital esophageal stenosis. *Laryngoscope, 79*(6), 1095–1104.

Dominguez, R., Zarabi, M., Oh, K. S., Bender, T. M., & Girdany, B. R. (1985). Congenital oesophageal stenosis. *Clinical Radiology, 36*(3), 263–266.

Easterling, C. (2015). *Esophageal disorders: What is the role of the speech pathologist?* Retrieved from https://dysphagiacafe.com/2015/02/05/esophageal-disorders-what-is-the-role-of-the-speech-pathologist/

Harrison, C. A., & Katon, R. M. (1992). Familial multiple congenital esophageal rings: Report of an affected father and son. *American Journal of Gastroenterology, 87*(12), 1813–1815.

Ibrahim, A. H., Al Malki, T. A., Hamza, A. F., & Bahnassy, A. F. (2007). Congenital esophageal stenosis associated with esophageal atresia: New concepts. *Pediatric Surgery International, 23*(6), 533–537.

Kim, S. H., Kim, H. Y., Jung, S. E., Lee, S. C., & Park, K. W. (2017). Clinical study of congenital esophageal stenosis: Comparison according to association of esophageal atresia and tracheoesophageal fistula. *Pediatric Gastroenterology, Hepatology, & Nutrition, 20*(2), 79–86.

Mai, C., Breysem, L., De Hertogh, G., Van Raemdonck, D., & Smet, M. H. (2015). An unusual presentation of congenital esophageal stenosis due to tracheobronchial remnants in a newborn prenatally diagnosed with duodenal atresia. *Journal of the Belgian Society of Radiology, 99*(2), 43–46. doi:http://doi.org/10.5334/jbr-btr.881

Michaud, L., Coutenier, F., Podevin, G., Bonnard, A., Becmeur, F., Khen-Dunlop, N., . . . Borderon, C. (2013). Characteristics and management of congenital esophageal stenosis: Findings from a multicenter study. *Orphanet Journal of Rare Diseases, 8*(1), 186.

Moore, K. L., & Persaud, T. V. N. (2003). *The developing human* (7th ed.). Philadelphia, PA: Elsevier.

Nihoule-Fekete, C., & Revillon, Y. (1987). Congenital oesophageal stenosis. A review of 20 cases. *Pediatric Surgery International, 2*, 86–89.

Nishina, T., Tsuchida, Y., & Saito, S. (1981). Congenital esophageal stenosis due to tracheobronchial remnants and its associated anomalies. *Journal of Pediatric Surgery, 16*(2), 190–193.

Ramesh, J. C., Ramanujam, T. M., & Jayaram, G. (2001). Congenital esophageal stenosis: Report of three cases, literature review, and a proposed classification. *Pediatric Surgery International, 17*(2–3), 188–192.

Rangel, R., & Lizarzabal, M. (1998). Familial multiple congenital esophageal rings. *Digestive Diseases (Basel, Switzerland), 16*(5), 325.

Romeo, E., Foschia, F., De Angelis, P., Caldaro, T., Di Abriola, G. F., Gambitta, R., . . . & Dall'Oglio, L. (2011). Endoscopic management of congenital esophageal stenosis. *Journal of Pediatric Surgery, 46*(5), 838–841.

Serrao, E., Santos, A., Gaivao, A., Tavares, A., & Ferreira, S. (2010). Congenital esophageal stenosis: A rare case of dysphagia. *Journal of Radiology Case Reports, 4*(6), 8.

Singh, A. P., Ansari, J. S., Gupta, P., Sharma, P., & Goyal, R. B. (2014). Congenital esophageal stenosis in an infant. *Journal of Evolution of Medical and Dental Sciences, 3*(38), 9820–9823.

Takamizawa, S., Tsugawa, C., Mouri, N., Satoh, S., Kanegawa, K., Nishijima, E., & Muraji, T. (2002). Congenital esophageal stenosis: Therapeutic strategy based on etiology. *Journal of Pediatric Surgery, 37*(2), 197–201.

Terui, K., Saito, T., Mitsunaga, T., Nakata, M., & Yoshida, H. (2015). Endoscopic management for congenital esophageal stenosis: A systematic review. *World Journal of Gastrointestinal Endoscopy, 7*(3), 183.

Vasudevan, S. A., Kerendi, F., Lee, H., & Ricketts, R. R. (2002). Management of congenital esophageal stenosis. *Journal of Pediatric Surgery, 37*(7), 1024–1026.

Yeung, C. K., Spitz, L., Brereton, R. J., Kiely, E. M., & Leake, J. (1992). Congenital esophageal stenosis due to tracheobronchial remnants: A rare but important association with esophageal atresia. *Journal of Pediatric Surgery, 27*(7), 852–855.

Younes, Z., & Johnson, D. A. (1999). Congenital esophageal stenosis: Clinical and endoscopic features in adults. *Digestive Diseases, 17*(3), 172–177.

Zhao, L. L., Hsieh, W. S., & Hsu, W. M. (2004). Congenital esophageal stenosis owing to ectopic tracheobronchial remnants. *Journal of Pediatric Surgery, 39*(8), 1183–1187.

5

Sporadic Inclusion Body Myositis

KEY WORDS: sporadic inclusion body myositis (sIBM), atrophy, cricopharyngeal myotomy, hypertonicity, dilatation, Mendelsohn maneuver

Definition

Sporadic inclusion body myositis (sIBM) also called inclusion body myositis (IBM) is a rare, debilitating, degenerative, and inflammatory disease in which aging appears to be the common denominator, as it usually occurs in patients older than 50 years of age. Sporadic inclusion body myositis is characterized by slow, progressive weakness and **atrophy** of the muscles of the limbs, face, and pharynx (Dalakas, 2015). The weakness and dysfunction of the pharyngeal and esophageal muscles often lead to the dysphagia that is a characteristic of sIBM. Dysphagia appears to be a major factor in the mortality of sIBM patients. An extensive study of 585 living and 149 deceased patients with sIBM carried out by Price et al. (2016) supported the finding that dysphagia contributed to a shorter life span in patients with sIBM. Sporadic inclusion body myositis is a complex, multifactorial disorder and the exact cause remains unclear. Askanas, Engel, and Nogalska (2015) found phenotypic similarities between sIMB muscle fibers and the brains of Alzheimer's and Parkinson's disease patients, diseases also associated with aging. It is interesting to note in the last two decades or so, sIBM is becoming less rare. Askanas et al. suggest physicians' greater awareness of the disease as well as more reliable pathologic markers may be responsible.

History

The term inclusion body myositis is a subtype of idiopathic inflammatory myositis. It was originally described by Yunis and Samaha (1971) in a case of myopathy that phenotypically suggested chronic polymyositis but showed cytoplasmic vacuoles and inclusions on muscle biopsy. In the subsequent years, sIBM has been increasingly recognized and reported, primarily because of increased awareness of the condition and improved histologic techniques.

It is clinically distinguished from other inflammatory myopathies by its selective pattern of muscle weakness and wasting, progressive clinical course, as well as pathologically by the combination of inflammatory and myodegenerative features with multiprotein aggregates in muscle tissue. Because of these unique phenotypic characteristics and the fact that the condition responds poorly to conventional forms of immune therapy, there is still much debate as to whether sIBM is a primary autoimmune disease of muscle or a degenerative myopathy with an associated vigorous immune response and secondary inflammatory component (Askanas et al., 2015; Needham & Mastaglia, 2007, 2008).

Etiology

The real cause of sIBM is largely unknown. Multiple immunological, genetic, environmental, as well as age-related factors play a significant role in the development of the disease. Sporadic inclusion body myositis is linked to two specific processes. One is autoimmune and the other is degenerative. Even though distinct, there is a possibility that these two processes are related.

According to NORD, some individuals with sIBM present with inflammatory white blood cells in the muscle tissue. This suggests that sIBM is an autoimmune disorder, hence, classified as such. Furthermore, the presence of an autoantigen in individuals with sIBM would appear to be confirmatory. In addition to the inflammatory condition, muscle tissue in sIBM appears to be degenerative. In actuality, the muscle tissue of some individuals with sIBM contains subcellular areas that have abnormal clusters of varied protein material. These clusters of protein are referred to as "inclusion bodies"; hence, the name of the disorder. In spite of these findings, it remains largely unclear what precipitates either the inflammatory or the degenerative processes present in sIBM.

Epidemiology

Sporadic inclusion body myositis affects males more often than females. According to NORD, the prevalence is estimated to lie somewhere between 10 to 71 persons per 1,000,000 in the general population. The onset typically is after 50 years of age. Even though sIBM is categorized as an orphan disease both in the United States and Europe, it is the most common muscle disease in older individuals (Needham, Mastaglia, & Garlepp, 2007), but its prevalence varies considerably across different populations and racial groups. The few epidemiological studies of sIBM suggest the variability of the disease in different population and ethnic groups.

The reported prevalence of sIBM varies from 4.7 million in the Netherlands to 14.9 million in Western Australia (Mastaglia, 2009) and may be underreported due to incomplete assessment or misdiagnosis (Needham et al., 2008). In the United States, the incidence of sIBM is more commonly reported on the East Coast, particularly in the New England state of Connecticut. Overall, prevalence in the general population ranges from 1 per 1,000,000 to about 1 per 14,000. Interestingly enough, there is an exponential increase when the population over 50 years of age is considered. Additionally, the current prevalence of sIBM appears to be higher than studies prior to 2015 may have reported. This rise in prevalence may be attributed to an increasing awareness of the disease as well as improvements in diagnostic criteria and study methodologies (Aoife et al., 2016).

Clinical Presentation

The clinical presentation of sIBM involves slow and steadily progressive muscle weakness. However, the severity, distribution, and progression of the muscle weakness vary across individuals. Some patients may present with one arm or leg more affected than the other. Generally, muscles of the thighs, wrists, and fingers are usually more affected than other muscles. Most patients with sIBM are at high fall risk. The muscle weakness that is pervasive in sIBM extends beyond involvement of the limbs. This weakness affects the muscles of the face, neck, and pharyngeal areas, thus leading to dysphagia.

Dysphagia is one of the phenotypes present in sIBM due to weakness of the pharyngeal muscles. According to Dimachkie and Barohn (2012), dysphagia can affect up to 70% of patients with sIBM. The nature of dysphagia in sIBM patients has not been specifically characterized. This may be because not all patients report the disorder, but may intuitively adjust their food textures. The onset of the dysphagia is insidious. Consequently, the early signs of the swallowing problem, such as mild coughing, may be overlooked and explained away as age related. Oh, Brumfield, Hoskin, Kasperbauer, and Basford (2008) reported up to 50% of sIBM patients exhibited debilitating dysphagia as the disease progressed. Not all patients present with the same type of dysphagia; however, choking is commonly reported secondary to upper esophageal sphincter weakness.

The mechanism of dysphagia in sIBM is similar to other types of inflammatory myopathies. There is inadequate pharyngeal contraction, poor relaxation of the cricopharyngeus muscle, and reduced hyolaryngeal elevation. Even so, not all patients will present with all of the above dysphagia manifestations in sIBM (Ko & Rubin, 2014).

Shibata et al. (2017) described an unusual case of a patient with sIBM whose only presenting symptom was dysphagia for at least 10 years before being officially diagnosed with sIBM. This patient developed progressive dysphagia, particularly for solid foods, and took a longer than usual time to complete meals. The dysphagia progressed to the point where the patient could no longer swallow. Results of a videofluoroscopic (VF) examination revealed upper esophageal sphincter (UES) dysfunction.

Esophageal dysfunction in sIBM patients has also been reported in other studies. One study by Murata, Kouda, Tajima, and Konda (2012) reported incomplete relaxation of the upper esophageal sphincter in all 10 patients studied. Cox et al. (2009) reported cricopharyngeal dysfunction in sIBM patients. Similar results were reported by Oh et al. (2007), who found oropharyngeal as well as cricopharyngeal dysfunction in the sIBM patients with dysphagia. On the other hand, Langdon, Mulcahy, Shepherd, Low, and Mastaglia (2012) analyzed the function of the upper esophageal sphincter (UES) for 214 swallows in 18 patients. Their results showed that contrary to the widely held belief of UES dysfunction in sIBM, the dysphagia was due to impaired muscle contraction and reduced hyolaryngeal excursion.

Management of Dysphagia

In sIBM, dysphagia is usually caused by weakness in the muscles of the throat in about a third of sufferers, and it usually occurs in greater than 60% of all cases. Patients with sIBM tend to show incomplete opening and pharyngeal muscle propulsion at the hypopharyngeal and upper esophageal sphincter (UES). Esophageal disorders are a common cause of morbidity and mortality in sIBM patients (Cherin et al., 2002). Treatment of dysphagia depends on the mechanism within the system that is impaired. For example, in many cases of sIBM, there may be tongue weakness, resulting in poor bolus control or decreased laryngeal elevation leading to penetration and aspiration of material. In a videofluoroscopic study of 43 cases of sIBM, Cox et al. (2009) reported 77% were found to have impaired propulsile function, 37% had cricopharyngeal sphincter dysfunction and impaired opening, and 53% had aspiration when swallowing fluids. Table 5–1 provides a list of some frequently impaired areas within the swallowing mechanism.

Many treatment options have been explored in the management of swallowing problems that accompany sIBM. These range from conservative measures such as dietary modifications, postural adjustments, and exercises provided by the speech-language pathologist to the more invasive approaches that involve pharmaceutical or surgical measures.

Not all of the traditional approaches to treating dysphagia secondary to a neurological problem have been successful with sIBM patients. The pervasive type of swallowing deficit in sIBM

Table 5–1. Some Common Areas of Impairment of the Swallowing Mechanism in sIBM

Common Impairments in the Swallowing Mechanism
Uncoordinated lingual movement
Reduced bolus control
Reduced tongue base retraction
Reduced laryngeal elevation
Reduced pharyngeal contraction
Residue of material on the posterior pharyngeal wall
Residue of material in the valleculae and pyriforms
Cricopharyngeal (UES) dysfunction
Penetration
Aspiration

appears to be a dysfunction of the UES. SLP intervention in most neurological cases of dysphagia favors the **Mendelsohn maneuver** (MM) (see Lazarus, 2013). The fact that MM is used to prolong the opening of the UES, thus creating more time for the passage of the bolus to the esophagus, makes it a viable option for managing dysphagia in sIBM. However, common approaches to the treatment of dysphagia in sIBM continue to be pharmaceutical and surgical, even though some are less successful than others; these will be discussed in the following sections.

Immunoglobulins and Corticosteroids

Cherin et al. (2002) reported that immunoglobulin either alone or with corticosteroids dramatically improved swallowing disorders. Unfortunately, to date, this method is still not proven to be an overall effective choice of treatment. Sporadic inclusion body myositis does not appear to respond to the immunosuppressive drugs or corticosteroids that are often used to treat inflammatory or autoimmune disorders. The primary goal of treatment from a gross motor perspective is to optimize muscle strength and to help the patient achieve his or her maximal function. It is believed that intravenous immunoglobulin may help some patients, but again, the benefits of this drug are short lived.

Botulinum Toxin

One innovative treatment proposed in the literature is the use of botulinum toxin. This may still be in the early stages of use. Schrey, Airas, Jokela, and Pulkkinen (2017) examined the effect of botulinum neurotoxin A (BoNT-A) to the cricopharyngeus muscle of patients with sIBM dysphagia. Schrey et al. reported that all 12 patients with cricopharyngeal dysfunction experienced normal swallow up to one year post final BoNT-A injection. There are sparse reports on this method of treating dysphagia in sIBM; clearly, this is an area that warrants further investigation.

Cricopharyngeal Myotomy

Cricopharyngeal myotomy is a surgical procedure in which the cricopharyngeal muscle from which the upper esophageal sphincter is derived is severed. According to Langdon et al. (2012), this procedure appears to be effective in managing dysphagia in some sIBM patients and more so when there is **hypertonicity** of the cricopharyngeus muscle. Hypertonicity contributes to the increased pressure in the cricopharyngeus region against which the pharyngeal constrictor muscles have to compete. Consequently, the goal in a cricopharyngeal myotomy is to decrease this pressure and allow flow, albeit passive, of material. In order for this procedure to be effective and safe, patients involved should have normal pharyngeal contraction (Murata et al., 2012). As promising as the cricopharyngeal myotomy procedure is for alleviating the upper esophageal sphincter (UES) dysfunction, Ko and Rubin (2014) admonish that this procedure should be reserved for those cases of sIBM in which conservative methods of managing the dysphagia have failed.

Pharyngoesophageal Dilatation

Pneumatic dilatation also known as balloon dilatation can be performed during endoscopy or fluoroscopy. In this procedure, a deflated balloon is inserted into the esophagus at the area that is narrow, and then it is inflated (Figure 5–1). Murata, Kouda, Tajima, and Kondo (2013) describe pharyngoesophageal **dilatation** in three sIBM patients with dysphagia. This procedure was performed three months after the patients were treated with intravenous immunoglobulin (IVIG). These researchers reported the elimination of the dysphagia, suggesting a possible treatment strategy for managing dysphagia in individuals. Parres (2015) reviewed cases of sIBM patients who were treated for dysphagia via alternative feeding (i.e., percutaneous endoscopic gastrostomy [PEG]), bougie upper esophageal dilatation with botuli-

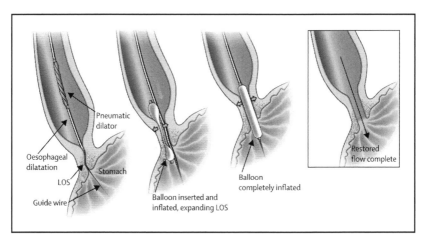

Figure 5–1. Esophageal dilatation. *Source*: From "Achalasia," by G. E. Boeckx-staens, G. Zaninotto, and J. E. Richter, 2014, *Lancet, 383*(9911), 83–93. doi.org /10.1016/S0140-6736(13)60651-0.

num neurotoxin A injection to the cricopharyngeus, and balloon dilatation of esophagus alone. Only the patients who had only balloon dilatation of the esophagus had longer-lasting subjective improvement of the dysphagia. This suggests the possibility of balloon dilatation as an effective symptomatic treatment for sIBM-associated dysphagia.

Mendelsohn Maneuver (MM)

The Mendelsohn maneuver (MM) is a noninvasive therapy approach frequently used by speech-language pathologists for patients with dysphagia. It is felt to be effective in volitionally prolonging the elevation of the larynx during the swallow, especially in patients who exhibit weak pharyngeal swallow. The premise of this technique is that the extent and the duration of laryngeal elevation would have a summative impact on the opening of the cricopharyngeus muscle. The technique is not curative for the

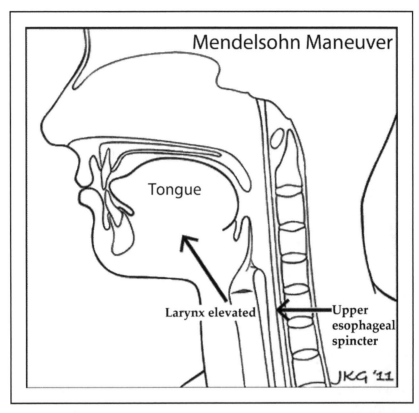

Figure 5–2. Illustration of the Mendelsohn maneuver. Adapted from "Mendelson maneuver and Masako maneuver," by C. Lazarus, in R. Shaker, C. Easterling, P. Belafsky, and G. Postma (Eds.), *Manual of Diagnostic and Therapeutic Techniques for Disorders of Deglutition*, 2013, by New York, NY: Springer.

dysphagia, but only serves to facilitate the movement of the larynx (Figure 5–2). One criterion essential for successful outcome of the MM is good physical condition. The MM requires increased muscular effort. The hallmark of sIBM is progressive muscle weakness; therefore, patients with this condition may not prove to be very successful candidates. A few earlier studies claim the usefulness of MM for helping some patients maintain a stable weight and continue eating without aspiration (Maugars et al., 1996; Oh et al., 2008). However, these studies did not provide information regarding the stage of sIBM or the severity of the dysphagia.

Summary

Sporadic inclusion body myositis is a rare, chronic, progressive, acquired disorder. It is distinguished by its selective muscle involvement that manifests itself in individuals over 50 years of age. Dysphagia commonly occurs in sIBM. In some cases, it may be the symptom that precedes the identification of the precipitating disease. The esophagus is often the most commonly affected and the most common source of the dysphagia. However, reduced pharyngeal contraction and hyolaryngeal elevation are also present. There is no known cure for sIBM, but management focuses on alleviating the presenting symptoms. Management options for dysphagia include diet modification and specific dysphagia exercises provided by a speech-language pathologist, drug therapy, esophageal dilatation, and cricopharyngeal myotomy.

References

Aoife, C., Capkun, G., Freitas, R., Vasanthaprasad, V., Ghosh, S., & Needham, M. (2016). Prevalence of sporadic inclusion body myositis. *Neurology, 86*(16 Suppl.), P1. 127.

Askanas, V., Engel, W. K., & Nogalska, A. (2015). Sporadic inclusion-body myositis: A degenerative muscle disease associated with aging, impaired muscle protein homeostasis and abnormal mitophagy. *Biochimica et Biophysica Acta (BBA)-Molecular Basis of Disease, 1852*(4), 633–643.

Cherin, P., Pelletier, S., Teixeira, A., Laforet, P., Genereau, T., Simon, A., . . . Herson, S. (2002). Results and long-term follow-up of intravenous immunoglobulin infusions in chronic, refractory polymyositis: An open study with thirty-five adult patients. *Arthritis & Rheumatism, 46*(2), 467–474.

Cherin, P., Pelletier, S., Teixeira, A., Laforet, P., Simon, A., Herson, S., & Eymard, B. (2002). Intravenous immunoglobulin for dysphagia of inclusion body myositis. *Neurology, 58*(2), 326–326.

Cox, F. M., Verschuuren, J. J., Verbist, B. M., Niks, E. H., Wintzen, A. R., & Badrising, U. A. (2009). Detecting dysphagia in inclusion body myositis. *Journal of Neurology, 256*(12).

Dalakas, M. C. (2015). Inflammatory muscle diseases. *New England Journal of Medicine, 372*(18), 1734–1747.

Dimachkie, M. M., & Barohn, R. J. (2012). Idiopathic inflammatory myopathies. *Seminars in Neurology, 32*(3), 227–236.

Ko, E. H., & Rubin, A. D. (2014). Dysphagia due to inclusion body myositis: Case presentation and review of the literature. *Annals of Otology, Rhinology, & Laryngology, 123*(9), 605–608.

Langdon, P. C., Mulcahy, K., Shepherd, K. L., Low, V. H., & Mastaglia, F. L. (2012). Pharyngeal dysphagia in inflammatory muscle diseases resulting from impaired suprahyoid musculature. *Dysphagia, 27*(3), 408–417.

Lazarus, C. (2013). Mendelson maneuver and Masako maneuver. In R. Shaker, C. Easterling, P. Belafsky, & G. Postma (Eds.), *Manual of diagnostic and therapeutic techniques for disorders of deglutition* (pp. 273–280). New York, NY: Springer.

Mastaglia, F. L. (2009). Sporadic inclusion body myositis: Variability in prevalence and phenotype and influence of the MHC. *Acta Myologica, 28*(2), 66.

Maugars, Y. M., Berthelot, J. M., Abbas, A. A., Mussini, J. M., Nguyen, J. M., & Prost, A. M. (1996). Long-term prognosis of 69 patients with dermatomyositis or polymyositis. *Clinical and Experimental Rheumatology, 14*(3), 263–274.

Murata, K. Y., Kouda, K., Tajima, F., & Kondo, T. (2012). A dysphagia study in patients with sporadic inclusion body myositis (s-IBM). *Neurological Sciences, 33*(4), 765–770.

Murata, K. Y., Kouda, K., Tajima, F., & Kondo, T. (2013). Balloon dilation in sporadic inclusion body myositis patients with dysphagia. *Clinical Medicine Insights: Case Reports, 6*, CCRep-S10200.

Needham, M., Corbett, A., Day, T., Christiansen, F., Fabian, V., & Mastaglia, F. L. (2008). Prevalence of sporadic inclusion body myositis and factors contributing to delayed diagnosis. *Journal of Clinical Neuroscience, 15*(12), 1350–1353.

Needham, M., & Mastaglia, F. L. (2007). Inclusion body myositis: current pathogenetic concepts and diagnostic and therapeutic approaches. *Lancet Neurology, 6*(7), 620–631.

Needham, M., & Mastaglia, F. L. (2008). Sporadic inclusion body myositis: A continuing puzzle. *Neuromuscular Disorders, 18*(1), 6–16.

Needham, M., Mastaglia, F. L., & Garlepp, M. J. (2007). Genetics of inclusion-body myositis. *Muscle & Nerve: Official Journal of the American Association of Electrodiagnostic Medicine, 35*(5), 549–561.

Oh, T. H., Brumfield, K. A., Hoskin, T. L., Kasperbauer, J. L., & Basford, J. R. (2008). Dysphagia in inclusion body myositis: Clinical features, management, and clinical outcome. *American Journal of Physical Medicine & Rehabilitation, 87*(11), 883–889.

Oh, T. H., Brumfield, K. A., Hoskin, T. L., Stolp, K. A., Murray, J. A., & Basford, J. R. (2007). Dysphagia in inflammatory myopathy: Clinical characteristics, treatment strategies, and outcome in 62 patients. *Mayo Clinic Proceedings, 82*(4), 441–447.

Parres, C. (2015). Pharyngoesophageal dilation and botulinum toxin therapy for dysphagia in patients with inclusion body myositis. *Neurology, 84*(14).

Price, M. A., Barghout, V., Benveniste, O., Christopher-Stine, L., Corbett, A., De Visser, M., . . . Mastaglia, F. (2016). Mortality and causes of death in patients with sporadic inclusion body myositis: Survey study based on the clinical experience of specialists in Australia, Europe and the USA. *Journal of Neuromuscular Diseases, 3*(1), 67–75.

Schrey, A., Airas, L., Jokela, M., & Pulkkinen, J. (2017). Botulinum toxin alleviates dysphagia of patients with inclusion body myositis. *Journal of the Neurological Sciences, 380*, 142–147.

Shibata, S., Izumi, R., Hara, T., Ohshima, R., Nakamura, N., Suzuki, N., . . . Aoki, M. (2017). Five-year history of dysphagia as a sole initial symptom in inclusion body myositis. *Journal of the Neurological Sciences, 381*, 325–327.

Yunis, E. J. & Samaha, X. (1971). Inclusion body myositis. *Laboratory Investigation, 25*(3), 557–577.

6

Moebius Syndrome

KEY WORDS: Moebius syndrome, extraocular, dysmorphism, cleft palate, brachydactyly, hypogonadism

Definition

According to the National Organization for Rare Diseases (NORD), **Moebius syndrome** (MBS), also known as congenital facial diplegia syndrome, is a rare, nonprogressive neurological disorder characterized by weakness or sometimes paralysis of multiple cranial nerves. Most individuals with MBS are born with complete facial paralysis and are unable to close their eyes or form facial expressions. Cranial nerves VI and VII—abducens and facial, respectively—are most often affected or even absent. The majority of studies refer to MBS as congenital facial weakness combined with abnormal ocular abduction. It appears that at the heart of this syndrome is the loss of function of the motor cranial nerves.

In their definition of MBS, the National Institute of Neurological Disorders and Stroke (NINDS) proposes that in addition to the involvement of CN VI and VII, other cranial nerves including CN III, CNV, CN IX, CN XI, and CN XII may also be affected (Table 6–1).

Table 6–1. Cranial Nerves Associated with Moebius Syndrome and Their Function

CRANIAL NERVES	FUNCTION
CN III (oculomotor)	Movement of the eyeball and eyelid
CN V (trigeminal)	Sensory and motor divisions; sensation to face; motor to lower jaw and ear; important for chewing
CN VI (abducens)	Lateral eyeball movement
CN VII (facial)	Facial expressions, tasting
CN VIII (vestibulocochlear/acoustic)	Cochlear or acoustic branch important for hearing; vestibular branch important for balance/equilibrium
CN IX (glossopharyngeal)	Tasting and swallowing
CN X (vagus)	Sensory to ear canal, pharynx, as well as digestive tract muscles involved in peristalsis, motor control of muscles in the throat
CN XI (accessory)	Controls muscles of neck for rotation, flexion, and extension of neck and shoulders
CN XII (hypoglossal)	Movement of the tongue

In 2007, the Moebius Syndrome Foundation Research Conference formally defined MBS as congenital, nonprogressive facial weakness with limited abduction of one or both eyes (Miller, 2007). Thus, facial weakness and ocular muscle weakness constitute the primary criteria for MBS. Additional features present in the disorder include hearing loss and other cranial nerve dysfunction, as well as motor, orofacial, musculoskeletal, neurodevelopmental, and social problems (Webb et al., 2012). The definition of and the diagnostic criteria for Moebius syndrome have not been without problems or controversy. The syndrome has been most often confused with hereditary congenital facial paresis (HCFP), which is restricted to involvement of the facial nerve and other abnormalities (Kniffin, 2016). After extensive studies of patients with Moebius syndrome, Verzijl, Van der Zwaag, Lammens, Ten Donkelaar, and Padberg (2005) concluded that HCFP and Moebius syndrome are not the same disorders, and furthermore, MBS is a complex disorder involving the brain stem. Verzijl et al. based their conclusions on MRI results of six of their patients with Moebius syndrome. These findings revealed abnormalities of the pons as well as the posterior fossa. Nevertheless, it is generally agreed that a striking feature of Moebius syndrome is the high incidence of accompanying congenital deformities.

History

Von Grafe first described congenital facial and abducens paralysis in the 1880s. Paul Julius Moebius, a German neurologist, then grouped the sixth and seventh nerve palsies into one syndrome (Moebius, 1888). Moebius described a rare neurological condition in a male patient who had no facial expression, no eye blink, and reduced lateral eye movements. Because of these findings, Moebius became the eponym to describe the disorder.

Moebius syndrome causes multiple abnormalities, hence it is known by other synonyms such as congenital facial diplegia, congenital oculofacial paralysis, MBS, and Moebius sequence. According to Palmer and Kao (2018), there is no single definition and diagnostic criteria for MBS among authors. However, for Von Graefe and Moebius, only those cases with congenital facial diplegia and bilateral abducens nerve palsies are confirmed cases of Moebius syndrome. Later, Henderson (1939) added congenital unilateral facial paralysis palsy as part of the diagnosis of MBS. He grouped the symptoms of MBS into three components: (1) facial diplegia with other cranial nerve palsies, (2) malformations particularly of the limbs, and (3) intellectual and developmental disabilities.

Etiology

The causes of MBS are poorly understood. However, most research-ers have proposed a multifactorial explanation for the syndrome. It is widely believed that the condition may be due to a com-bination of genetic, environmental, neurological, and vascular factors.

It is generally accepted that there may be a genetic basis in a subset of patients, but these cases are sporadic (Verzijl et al., 2005). In the familial patterns of MBS, there is some evidence that the disorder is inherited as an autosomal dominant trait.

Occurrences of maternal trauma may result in impaired or interrupted blood flow or oxygen (hypoxia) to the developing fetus. Intrauterine toxic exposure, certain medications taken during pregnancy, as wells drugs such as cocaine may also be risk factors for Moebius syndrome. For example, misoprostol, also known by the brand name Cytotec, is used to induce labor and has a high success rate (90% success with 10% failure). Studies show that the use of misoprostol during pregnancy increases the risk of MBS (Koren & Schuler, 2001).

The neurological basis for MBS proposes that cranial nerves VI through XII are involved. The facial nerve, CN VII, is involved in all cases; and the abducens, CN VI, is involved in approximately 75% of MBS cases (National Organization for Rare Disorders, 2019). Some researchers suggest MBS may be due to agenesis of the cranial nerve nuclei. Manifested symptoms of MBS are most likely related to incomplete development of the cranial nerves and other parts of the central nervous system.

Epidemiology

In 2007, the Moebius Foundation estimated that there were approx-imately 2,000 cases of MBS worldwide (Broussard & Borazjani, 2008). However, the exact incidence is unknown, even though researchers estimate the condition can be 1 in 50,000 to 1 in 500,000 babies in the United States. MBS appears to affect males and females in equal numbers (National Organization for Rare Diseases, 2019). Most cases are sporadic, but there are documented familial cases representing about 2% (Picciolini et al., 2016.)

Clinical Presentation

MBS, as described elsewhere in this chapter, is a rare neurological condition. The primary presenting symptoms are unilateral or bilateral facial paralysis and defective **extraocular** eye movements. These presentations are secondary to defects of cranial nerves VII and VI, respectively. In addition to these classic features of the syndrome, underdevelopment of cranial nerves XII (hypoglossal), V (trigeminal), IX (glossopharyngeal), and X (vagus) is also present. A multiplicity of deformities and conditions may accompany MBS. Some patients present with craniofacial **dysmorphisms** such as mandibular hypoplasia, microstomia, temporomandibular jaw dysfunction, **cleft palate**, and external ear deformities, as well as limb and musculoskeletal malformations (syndactyly, **brachydactyly**, or absent digits and talipes) and eye abnormalities such as inability to blink or to move eyeballs from side to side. In some cases, other associated disorders including, seizures, cardiac diseases, hypogonadism, and intellectual dysfunction may be present (see Table 6–2 for clinical features of MBS).

Poor oral muscle coordination in newborns with MBS causes inability to suck. This frequently leads to decreased feedings. The condition appears related to involvement of CN IX and X and may be associated with the dysphagia commonly associated with MBS (see Table 6–2).

Dysphagia in MBS

Children with MBS may have difficulty sucking soon after birth. This can lead to poor nutrition, and in most cases, aspiration. Frequent aspiration can lead to aspiration pneumonia.

Table 6–2. Clinical Synopsis of Moebius Syndrome

Head & Neck	Effects
Face	Bilateral paresis Micrognathia (64% of patients)
Ears	External ear defects (47% of patients)
Eyes	Bilateral abduction & adduction palsy, hypertelorism (25% of patients) Duane retraction syndrome (34% of patients) Epicanthal folds (89% of patients)
Nose	Flattened nasal bridge (81% of patients)
Mouth	High-arched palate (61% of patients) Tongue hypoplasia (77% of patients) Limited tongue movement Unilateral tongue weakness Bifid uvula (11% of patients) Absent jaw rotation
Teeth	Dentition defects (37% of patients)
Abdomen	Feeding problems in infancy Dysphagia
Neurologic (CNS)	Delayed motor development Hypotonia in infancy Language delay (55% of patients) Dysarthria Facial nerve palsy (CN VII) Abducens nerve palsy (CN VI) Clumsiness (82% of patients) Poor coordination (83% of patients) Dysdiadochokinesis (63% of patients)
(PNS)	Loss of sensation on the face (CN V) (11% of patients)

Since individuals with MBS present with multiple facial and oral deficits such as high arch palate, lingual hypoplasia, reduced tongue movement, unilateral tongue movement, inability to achieve mouth closure, absent rotary jaw movement, and poor dentition, swallowing problems are inevitable. Dibin, John, Annapoorani, and Abraham (2017) cited the facial and oral deficits noted previously as classic symptoms of Moebius syndrome and risk factors for aspiration pneumonia.

There are characteristic features of MBS that in combination may lead to a larger deficit. For example, the limited mouth opening, inadequate coughing and swallowing reflexes, and aspiration further contribute to respiratory problems (Budić, Šurdilović, Slavković, Marjanović, Stević, & Simić, 2016). Budić et al. reported a case of a 10-year-old female with MBS who had multiple clinical expressions typical of MBS as well as other unusual, progressive clinical manifestations that led to severe airway challenges, thus complicating management of her dysphagia symptoms.

Management of Dysphagia

There is no known cure for MBS; hence, management for individuals with the disorder takes the form of supportive care based on the presenting symptoms. Intervention requires a multidisciplinary diagnostic protocol. This should take the form of interviews with parents or the caregivers in order to establish a thorough medical and genetic history. There should be pediatric assessments including physical and occupational therapy so that the skills and functional development of the child can be ascertained for the purposes of prognosis and treatment. Since swallowing is a critical part of the management of dysphagia, the speech-language pathologist will play a vital role in management. Dysphagia and the aspiration that may result are the most life-threatening problems patients with MBS encounter (Ha & Messieha, 2003).

MBS is not progressive. However, infants may require feeding tubes or adaptive feeding bottles to facilitate adequate nutrition. Inability to maintain or even achieve lip closure is a common characteristic of MBS. The feeding problems experienced by children with MBS are largely sucking–swallowing difficulty, respiratory problems, and decreased sensitivity of the orofacial area.

Some children may have paralysis, while others may experience paresis.

Paralysis is defined as complete loss of motor function as well as sensation. Paresis, on the other hand, may affect the muscle motion but not the sensation. For those children with paralysis, the goal may be to teach compensatory motor skills; whereas in paresis, the goal will be to improve the functional capacity of the affected muscles.

Improving upper lip strength and mobility is one of the main goals for children with MBS (Rosenfeld-Johnson, 1999). In terms of breastfeeding, drinking from a bottle or cup, removing food from the spoon, or propelling the food over the tongue, adequate lip mobility is required. In many cases, feeding is rendered extremely difficult; therefore, the child has to be fed via feeding tubes.

Not only are swallowing and feeding impacted in MBS, but a wide spectrum of functional abilities is also affected. The difficulties in management create much hardship on the mother as well as the child. For one thing, the lack of facial communicative expressions and difficulties in producing speech sounds negatively affect the reward of the parent–child feedback interaction, thus leading to a failure of mother–child attachment (Picciolini et al., 2016).

The International Classification of Functioning Disability and Health: Children and Youth (ICF-CY) that was instituted by the World Health Organization (WHO) has devised a standard of care for describing functioning, disability, and health. The ICF-CY is particularly suited for the child with MBS for the following reasons:

1. The visual deficits in MBS inhibit the child's recognition of things and activities in the world, thus language skills are impaired.

2. The primary motor problems interfere with movement, and all aspects of feeding.

3. Secondary deficits are manifested in the inability to recognize facial expressions. This can lead to a failure to develop socialization skills.

The ICF-CY framework for describing functions, activities, and participation—once known as impairment, disability, and handicap, respectively—allows the rehabilitation team to identify the various complexities of ailments seen in children with MBS and manage each aspect from a holistic perspective, as Figure 6–1 outlines. This framework offers an important guide to rehabilitation

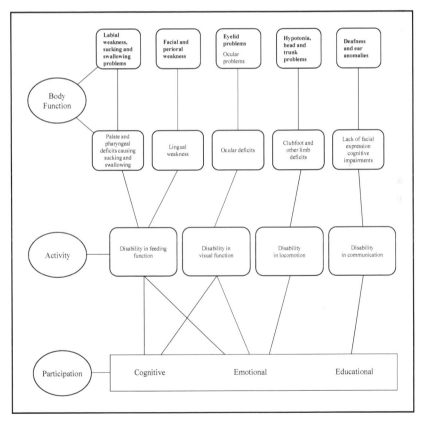

Figure 6–1. ICF-CY Framework of function, activity, and participation (ICF-CY = International Classification of Functioning, Disability and Health: Children and Youth).

from a multidisciplinary perspective, thus providing the optimum care for both child and caregiver.

Summary

Mobius syndrome is a rare, congenital condition that is characterized by the absence or the underdevelopment of the abducens nerve (CN VI) and facial nerve (CN VII), even though other cranial nerves may also be involved. The etiology is multifactorial. Several theories have been proposed. The most accepted are transient ischemic or hypoxic insult to the fetus, infections, and genetic. MBS has an estimated incidence of 1 in 100,000 births. This clinical syndrome was first described by the German neurologist Paul Julius Mobius (1853–1907). The earliest clinical signs of the disorder are the inability of the newborn to suckle, an expressionless face, and marked drooling. Paralysis may be unilateral or bilateral. Since the disorder is multifactorial, the best approach to treatment is from a multidisciplinary team approach. The primary problem is that of sucking and swallowing; therefore, treatment initially focuses on nutrition. Most infants will be fed via tube feedings until they are able to support themselves through independent oral feeding.

References

Broussard, A. B., & Borazjani, J. G. (2008). The faces of Moebius syndrome: Recognition and anticipatory guidance. *American Journal of Maternal/Child Nursing, 33*(5), 272–278.

Budić, I., Šurdilović, D., Slavković, A., Marjanović, V., Stević, M., & Simić, D. (2016). Moebius syndrome: Challenges of airway management. *Acta Clinica Croatica, 55*(Suppl. 1), 94–97.

Dibin, R., John, B., Annapoorani, & Abraham, A. A. (2017). Moebius syndrome: Oromandibular-limb hypogenesis spectrum—a case report. *International Journal of Science and Research, 6*(2). doi: 10.21275/ART2017878.

Ha, C. Y., & Messieha, Z. S. (2003). Management of a patient with Mobius syndrome: A case report. *Special Care in Dentistry, 23*(3), 111–116.

Henderson, J. L. (1939). The congenital facial diplegia syndrome. Clinical features, pathology and aetiology. A review of sixty-one cases. *Brain, 62*, 381–403.

Kniffin, C. (2016). Moebius syndrome. Online Mendelian Inheritance in Man. Retrieved from https://www.omim.org/entry/157900

Koren, G., & Schuler, L. (2001). Taking drugs during pregnancy. How safe are the unsafe? *Canadian Family Physician, 47*(5), 951–953.

Miller, G. (2007). Neurological disorders. The mystery of the missing smile. *Science, 316*, 826–827.

Moebius, P. J. (1888). Ueber angeborene doppelseitige abducens facialis lahmung. *Munch. Medi. Wochenschr., 35*, 108–111.

National Organization for Rare Disorders. (2019). Retrieved from https://rarediseases.org/rare-diseases/moebius-syndrome/

Palmer, C. A., & Kao, A. (2018). *Mobius syndrome clinical presentation.* Retrieved February 23, 2012, from http://emedicine.medscape.com.

Picciolini, O., Porro, M., Cattaneo, E., Castelletti, S., Masera, G., Mosca, F., & Bedeschi, M. F. (2016). Moebius syndrome: Clinical features, diagnosis, management and early intervention. *Italian Journal of Pediatrics, 42*(1), 56.

Rosenfeld-Johnson, S. (1999). Improving feeding safety and speech clarity in clients with Moebius syndrome. Retrieved April 16, 2008.

Verzijl, H. T., Van der Zwaag, B., Lammens, M., Ten Donkelaar, H. J., & Padberg, G. W. (2005). The neuropathology of hereditary congenital facial palsy vs Möbius syndrome. *Neurology, 64*(4), 649–653.

Webb, B. D., Shaaban, S., Gaspar, H., Cunha, L. F., Schubert, C. R., Hao, K., . . . Oystreck, D. T. (2012). HOXB1 founder mutation in humans recapitulates the phenotype of Hoxb1–/– mice. *American Journal of Human Genetics, 91*(1), 171–179.

7

Ataxia Telangiectasia

KEY WORDS: ataxia, Louis-Bar syndrome, immunodeficiency, cerebellar ataxia, bronchopulmonary

Definition

Ataxia telangiectasia (AT) or **Louis-Bar syndrome** is a rare, progressive, monogenic neurodegenerative disease with a pattern of autosomal recessive inheritance. Ataxia, **immunodeficiency**, sinopulmonary infections, premature aging, nutritional compromise, and oropharyngeal dysphagia are major characteristics of AT.

Ataxia refers to poor coordination or lack of order. Onset occurs in infancy and becomes more apparent as the child begins to walk, and the disease is relentlessly progressive. Ataxia at this stage is associated with abnormal head movements.

Telangiectasia refers to small-dilated blood vessels usually occurring at the corners of the eyes or on the surface of the ears and cheeks. These signs are more noticeable after 3 to 6 years of age or during adolescence. Both the ataxia and the telangiectasia are the hallmarks of the disease. Speech and swallowing problems are also markedly present. Gastrostomy tube (GT) feedings are commonly used to manage the dysphagia with concomitant aspiration. AT is a symptom of cerebellar dysfunction. The term *ataxia* means without order. **Cerebellar ataxia** causes incoordination of movements because of lesions in the afferent and efferent cerebellar connections (Chakor & Bharote, 2012).

History

The earliest reports describing patients who fit the profile of AT date as far back as the mid-1950s when Boder and Sedgwick (1958) proposed the term ataxia telangiectasia. The syndrome was named ataxia telangiectasia because of the two remarkable features, cerebellar ataxia and conjunctival telangiectasia. However, other designations were ascribed to the disorder; these include Louis-Bar syndrome, suggested by Centerwall and Miller (1958), as well as Boder-Sedgwick syndrome, proposed by Sagarra in 1959 (Sedgwick & Boder (1991). The eponym Louis-Bar was based on the findings of Madame Louis-Bar, a Belgian neurologist who described a 9-year-old male with progressive cerebellar ataxia with cutaneous telangiectasia. Consequently, ataxia telangiectasia was known as Louis-Bar syndrome for many years until Boder and Sedgwick described the clinical as well as pathologic features of AT, hence the name (Boder, 1975; Boder & Sedgwick, 1970).

Etiology

AT is an inherited autosomal recessive trait. One gene received from the father and one gene received from the mother determine a genetic disease. A recessive genetic disorder occurs when the person inherits the same abnormal gene for the same trait from each parent (National Organization for Rare Diseases, 2019). In the case of AT, mutations in the ATM gene are at the heart of the disorder. The role of the ATM gene is to provide instructions for making a protein that facilitates cell division and DNA repair. The protein is also critical to the normal development and activity of several body systems such as the nervous system and the immune system. Any mutations in the ATM gene will either reduce or completely dissolve the function of the ATM protein, causing cells to die. For example, cells in the cerebellum—the part of the brain responsible for coordinating movements—are particularly affected when there is a loss of the ATM protein. This is precisely the case in Ataxia telangiectasia. Furthermore, the impaired gene causing AT is located on the long arm (q) of chromosome 11 (11q22.3). Chromosomes, which are in the nucleus of all body cells, carry the genetic characteristics of all individuals. Each chromosome has a short arm called "p" and a long arm identified as "q." Under normal circumstances, the protein known as ATM is an enzyme that responds to DNA damage by triggering the accumulation of another protein that prevents cells from dividing. This is the tumor suppressor protein. On the other hand, in persons with AT, the abnormal mutations of the ATM gene prevent the accumulation of the protein causing cells with DNA damage to continue to proliferate abnormally, thus increasing the risk for cancer development.

Epidemiology

Ataxia telangiectasia occurs in all regions of the world, with an estimated incidence of about 1in 40,000 to 1 in 100,000 births (Rothblum-Oviatt et al., 2016). Broides et al. (2017) reported the frequency of AT to be significantly higher in the consanguineous relationships that frequently occur in the Bedouin population in southern Israel. However, it is difficult to diagnose before the patient reaches the age of 2 years, unless the disease is already present in the family (Rondon-Melo, de Almeida, de Andrade, Sassi, & Molini-Avejonas, 2017).

AT is reported in all races, but mortality rates are different across ethnic groups. However, the disorder occurs equally between males and females. There are no characteristic age-related features of the disorder. However, ataxia, which is usually the first diagnostic hallmark, is seen in the early years. After the age of 5, the progression of the ataxia is readily apparent, and by the time the child reaches prepubescent years, he or she may require a wheelchair (Trimis, Athanassaki, Kanariou, & Giannoulia-Karantana, 2004). Death typically occurs in early to late adolescence, usually from **bronchopulmonary** infection. However, in the absence of bronchopulmonary disease, patients may survive well into the fifth or sixth decade.

Clinical Presentation

In the classic presentation of AT, ataxia first appears during the toddler stage when the child begins to sit and walk. The myriad of features present in AT can vary among individuals as well present at different ages. Some common features of AT are ataxia, oculomotor apraxia, telangiectasia, cancer, delayed hormonal development, diabetes, dysarthria, and oropharyngeal dysphagia. A detailed list of common features is displayed in Table 7–1. The discussion in this section will center around the dysphagia symptoms in AT.

Dysphagia

Dysphagia, particularly oropharyngeal, is common and progressive in individuals with ataxia telangiectasia and tends to worsen with age (Lefton-Greif et al., 2000). The literature also describes impaired swallowing and its association with pulmonary disease in individuals with AT. The typical swallowing symptoms displayed in AT are coughing, choking during the swallow, and incoordination between breathing and swallowing—all leading to aspiration (Lefton-Greif et al., 2000).

Table 7–1. Common Features of Ataxia Telangiectasia

Feature	Description
Ataxia	Difficulty with control of movement
Oculomotor apraxia	Difficulty with coordination of eye movement
Telangiectasia	Dilated blood vessels of sclera of the eyes and of the skin
Speech	Slurred/distorted speech sounds
Swallowing problems	Drooling, choking, prolonged mealtimes, aspiration pneumonia
Nystagmus	Rapid involuntary eye movement
Motor	Increasing incoordination of arms and hands
Dyspnea	Disease of cardiac muscle characterized by shortness of breath upon exertion
Polydipsia	Abnormal increase in thirst
Polyuria	Abnormal increase in urination

In AT, most dysphagic problems typically emerge during the second decade of life (Crawford et al., 2000). Unlike most neuromuscular disorders, the underlying cause of the dysphagia tends to be muscular discoordination rather than primary weakness. The ataxia and bulbar dysfunction present in AT are most likely responsible for the discoordination of oral motor and general swallowing movements. Most neuromuscular patients tend to have swallowing problems with thicker viscosities of liquids as well as with solid textures because of a weak swallow (van den Engel-Hoek et al., 2014). On the other hand, individuals with AT tend to have problems with thin consistencies, as reported by modified barium swallow studies (Lefton-Greif et al., 2000), but these studies were carried out with older patients drinking through a straw.

According to studies reviewed by Bhatt et al. (2015), fatigue is characteristic of patients with AT and may be a contributor to the inefficient cough and aspiration present in many of these patients. It is noteworthy that the onset of dysphagia in this population appears to coincide with the decrease in nutritional status, even though it is not to be definitively ascertained that the dysphagia is the cause or effect.

Since ataxia is defined by "lack of order," disruption in movement or coordination is a prominent feature. Disruptions in the temporal relationships between breathing and swallowing are associated with the oropharyngeal dysphagia characteristic of AT (Lefton-Greif, Perlman, He, Lederman, & Crawford, 2016). However, to appreciate fully why this occurs, it is important to understand the close correspondence between the pathways for air and food. Swallowing and respiration are highly coordinated in adult humans (Matsuo & Palmer, 2009). Anatomically, the feeding process and breathing process share the same structures. The pharynx is the route for both swallowing and breathing, even though it is used differently for each activity. According to Matsuo and Palmer (2009), in adult humans, swallowing usually starts during the expiratory phase of breathing, and respiration resumes with continued expiration after swallowing. The predominant respiration–swallowing pattern in healthy adult humans is the "exhale—swallow—exhale" (E-Sw-E) pattern followed by "inhale—swallow—exhale" (I-Sw-E) pattern (Matsuo & Palmer, 2009). On the other hand, the E-Sw-E and "inhale—swallow—inhale" (I-Sw-I) patterns tend to occur rarely in the healthy adult swallow. It turns out that the resumption of exhalation after the swallow serves as a physiological airway protection mechanism because it can prevent inhalation of residual material left in the pharynx after swallowing. Lefton-Greif et al. (2016) demonstrated that this pattern of swallow, the E-Sw-E, is the safest and commonly occurs in healthy individuals regardless of age. However, individuals with AT tend to exhibit the unsafe I-Sw-I pattern more frequently than healthy adults.

Management of Dysphagia

Dysphagia is common in AT and typically becomes more apparent after the second decade of life. This difficulty swallowing occurs because of the neurological changes that interfere with the coordinated movements of the mouth and pharynx that are vital for safe, efficient swallowing. The discoordination of the oral musculature may lead to difficulty masticating. Discoordination of the pharynx may contribute to aspiration of foods and liquids. These difficulties result in the prolongation of the meal, poor nutrition, and more importantly, serious pulmonary deficits.

The goal of managing swallowing difficulties in AT is to facilitate safe, adequate nutrition and hydration. Since AT is a degenerative condition, dysphagia intervention is required at various stages of the progression of the disease.

Unfortunately, there is currently no cure for AT and there is no known way to slow the progression of the disease. Consequently, treatment for the most part is supportive and proactive. According to Vogel, Keage, Johnsson, and Schalling (2015), management approaches are based on the mode of delivery, including direct and indirect approaches, compensatory techniques, and, in most cases, alternative feeding.

Direct Approach

This approach is safer with those patients who have good cognition and are still able to feed themselves orally when given facilitating instructions. In this method, the patient is able to eat specific types of foods and liquids while being taught a particular exercise or strategy aimed at improving a safer swallow. Some of these strategies and exercises can range from utilizing a chin down posture during the swallow to an effortful swallow tactic—all aimed at mechanically facilitating a safe swallow.

Indirect Approach

The purpose of the indirect method of treatment is to strengthen and improve coordination of structures, wherever possible, in order to promote safety in the swallow. Based on the work by Sciortino, Liss, Case, Gerritsen, and Katz (2003), the indirect method of treating can include oral motor exercises, diet modification, as well as tactile thermal stimulation techniques.

Compensatory Techniques

Compensatory strategies such as postural adjustments and special utensils are useful to accommodate the movement disorder associated with the ataxia. These strategies include postural modification such as altered head position, the use of special utensils such as controlled-flow lids, and modified seating.

Alternative Feeding

Gastrostomy tube (GT) feedings are employed to manage dysphagia in patients with AT, specifically those who are at high risk for aspiration or failure to thrive (Lefton-Greif, Crawford, McGrath-Morrow, Carson, & Lederman, 2011). Based on their retrospective study of patients with gastrostomy tubes secondary to AT, Lefton-Greif et al. concluded that AT patients tend to tolerate GT more easily when it is placed early in the progression of the disease. Specifically, patients with childhood onset of swallowing disorders tend to glean more benefit from early placement versus later placement of the GT feeding tubes. Feeding tubes in general may also serve to provide adequate caloric intake without the stress and time commitment of prolonged meals. GTs do not prevent oral feedings, but may serve as the main source of caloric intake in the nutritionally fragile patient who can still eat small amounts orally (Rothblum-Oviatt et al., 2016).

Summary

Ataxia telangiectasia (AT) is a rare, neurodegenerative disease that is characterized by ataxia, immunodeficiency, sino-pulmonary infections, premature aging, nutritional compromise, and dysphagia. It is an inherited, autosomal recessive trait. Ataxia refers to poor coordination and telangiectasia refers to small-dilated blood vessels; the hallmarks of the disease. Symptoms often appear in early childhood when the child is beginning to walk. Speech and swallowing problems are prominent features of the disorder. Gastrostomy tube feedings are commonly used to manage the dysphagia. AT occurs in all races, but mortality rates are different across ethnic groups. However, the disorder occurs equally between males and females. Currently, there is no cure for this disease. While the mortality rate tends to be common in the second decade of life, there has been some cases of survival in the sixth and seventh decades.

References

Bhatt, J. M., Bush, A., van Gerven, M., Nissenkorn, A., Renke, M., Yarlett, L., . . . Zinna, S. (2015). ERS statement on the multidisciplinary respiratory management of ataxia telangiectasia. *European Respiratory Review, 24*(138), 565–581.

Boder, E. (1975). Ataxia-telangiectasia: Some historic, clinical and pathologic observations. *Birth Defects Original Article Series, 11*(1), 255–270.

Boder, E., & Sedgwick, R. P. (1958). Ataxia-telangiectasia: A familial syndrome of progressive cerebellar ataxia, oculocutaneous telangiectasia and frequent pulmonary infection. *Pediatrics, 21*(4), 526–554.

Boder, E., & Sedgwick, R. P. (1970). Ataxia-telangiectasia (clinical and immunological aspects). *Psychiatrie, Neurologie und medizinische Psychologie. Beihefte, 13*, 8–16.

Broides, A., Nahum, A., Mandola, A. B., Rozner, L., Pinsk, V., Ling, G., . . . Givon-Lavi, N. (2017). Incidence of typically severe primary immunodeficiency diseases in consanguineous and non-consanguineous populations. *Journal of Clinical Immunology, 37*(3), 295–300.

Centerwall, W. R., & Miller, M. M. (1958). Ataxia, telangiectasia, and sinopulmonary infections: A syndrome of slowly progressive deterioration in childhood. *AMA Journal of Diseases of Children, 95*(4), 385–396.

Chakor, R. T., & Bharote, H. (2012). Inherited ataxia with slow saccades. *Journal of Postgraduate Medicine, 58*(4), 318.

Crawford, T. O., Mandir, A. S., Lefton-Greif, M. A., Goodman, S. N., Goodman, B. K., Sengul, H., & Lederman, H. M. (2000). Quantitative neurologic assessment of ataxia-telangiectasia. *Neurology, 54*(7), 1505–1509.

Lefton-Greif, M. A., Crawford, T. O., McGrath-Morrow, S., Carson, K. A., & Lederman, H. M. (2011). Safety and caregiver satisfaction with gastrostomy in patients with ataxia telangiectasia. *Orphanet Journal of Rare Diseases, 6*(1), 23.

Lefton-Greif, M. A., Crawford, T. O., Winkelstein, J. A., Loughlin, G. M., Koerner, C. B., Zahurak, M., & Lederman, H. M. (2000). Oropharyngeal dysphagia and aspiration in patients with ataxia-telangiectasia. *The Journal of Pediatrics, 136*(2), 225–231.

Lefton-Greif, M. A., Perlman, A. L., He, X., Lederman, H. M., & Crawford, T. O. (2016). Assessment of impaired coordination between respiration and deglutition in children and young adults with ataxia telangiectasia. *Developmental Medicine & Child Neurology, 58*(10), 1069–1075.

Matsuo, K., & Palmer, J. B. (2009). Coordination of mastication, swallowing and breathing. *Japanese Dental Science Review, 45*(1), 31–40.

National Organization for Rare Diseases. (2019). *Ataxia Telangiectasia.* Retrieved from https://rarediseases.org/rare-diseases/ataxia-telangiectasia/

Rondon-Melo, S., de Almeida, I. J., de Andrade, C. R. F., Sassi, F. C., & Molini-Avejonas, D. R. (2017). Ataxia telangiectasia in siblings: Oral motor and swallowing characterization. *American Journal of Case Reports, 18*, 783.

Rothblum-Oviatt, C., Wright, J., Lefton-Greif, M. A., McGrath-Morrow, S. A., Crawford, T. O., & Lederman, H. M. (2016). Ataxia telangiectasia: A review. *Orphanet Journal of Rare Diseases, 11*(1), 159.

Sciortino, K. F., Liss, J. M., Case, J. L., Gerritsen, K. G., & Katz, R. C. (2003). Effects of mechanical, cold, gustatory, and combined stimulation to the human anterior faucial pillars. *Dysphagia, 18*(1), 16–26.

Sedgwick, R. P., & Boder, E. (1991). *Handbook of Clinical Neurology. Hereditary Neuropathies and Spinocerebellar Atrophies.* Amsterdam, The Netherlands: Elsevier Science Publishers.

Trimis, G. G., Athanassaki, C. K., Kanariou, M. M., & Giannoulia-Karantana, A. A. (2004). Unusual absence of neurologic symptoms in a six-year old girl with ataxia-telangiectasia. *Journal of Postgraduate Medicine, 50*(4), 270.

van den Engel-Hoek, L., Erasmus, C. E., van Hulst, K. C., Arvedson, J. C., de Groot, I. J., & de Swart, B. J. (2014). Children with central and peripheral neurologic disorders have distinguishable patterns of dysphagia on videofluoroscopic swallow study. *Journal of Child Neurology, 29*(5), 646–653.

Vogel, A. P., Keage, M. J., Johansson, K., & Schalling, E. (2015). Treatment for dysphagia (swallowing difficulties) in hereditary ataxia. *Cochrane Database of Systematic Reviews*, (11).

8

Pontocerebellar Hypoplasia

KEY WORDS: pontocerebellar hypoplasia, microcephaly, extra-pyramidal dyskinesia, Purkinje cells, chorea, athetosis, dystonia

Definition

Pontocerebellar hypoplasia (PCH) describes a heterogeneous group of neurodegenerative disorders with a prenatal onset. These disorders tend to affect the cerebellum and the pons, although earlier reports have identified spinal motor neurodegeneration, also known as spinal muscular atrophy (Norman & Urich, 1960; van Dijk, Baas, Barth, & Poll-The, 2018). There are several variants of PCH. Namavar and colleagues (2011) described seven different subtypes (PCH1–7) all sharing common characteristics such as atrophy of the cerebellum and pons (hypoplasia), progressive **microcephaly**, and various cerebral involvement, including cognitive and motor involvements as well as seizures.

The most current updates on PCH (van Dijk et al., 2018) have identified 11 types, and a further 17 PCH-related genes are now listed on the official site of the Online Mendelian Inheritance in Man (OMIN) database. However, Barth (1993) first classified PCH into two subtypes: PCH1 and PCH2. PCH1 was characterized by

97

anterior horn degeneration in the spinal cord with muscle weakness and hypotonia. PCH2, on the other hand, was distinguished by neonatal jitteriness, incoordination of sucking and swallowing disorders, impaired voluntary motor development, and marked cognitive deficits. This chapter will focus on PHC2 because of the presence of dysphagia.

History

The main feature of PCH is the pontocerebellar hypoplasia. The first identification of a child with underdevelopment of the pons and cerebellum was publicized in the early 1900s. Later, Krause (1929) described clinical features associated with PCH when he reported a 16-month-old child with spasticity microcephaly and dysphagia.

Over the last 20 years, more information has emerged on PCH. Most notable was the isolation of the gene that causes PCH in a cluster of families in the Netherlands. Barth, Vrensen, Uylings, Oorthuys, and Stam (1990) described seven young children from related families who presented with microcephaly, spastic pareses, severe **extra-pyramidal dyskinesia**, and failure to acquire any voluntary skills. CT scans of these patients revealed severe pontocerebellar hypoplasia and cerebral atrophy, with more loss of neurons in the pons and cerebellum compared to other brain regions (Eggens, 2016). Even though many subtypes of PHC have been identified, the latest count registering at 11 (van Dijk et al., 2018), they all share commonalities of hypoplasia and/or atrophy of the cerebellum and pons, fetal onset of the disease, and severe developmental delays with significantly reduced cognitive and motor skills (Eggens, 2016). Apparently, the reason for the small size of the pons and cerebellum is due to the loss of **Purkinje cells**, which are essential to the body's motor function, fragmentation of the dentate nucleus, and loss of the pontine nuclei. Even with the common features of the different subtypes of PCH, each subtype still exhibits distinct clinical characteristics (Table 8–1).

Table 8–1. Common Features of PCH

Medical Terms
Cerebral atrophy
Cerebral cortical atrophy
Cortical gyral simplification
Death in childhood
Ventriculomegaly
Abnormality of the periventricular white matter
Autosomal recessive inheritance
Babinski sign
Cerebellar atrophy
Cerebellar hemisphere hypoplasia
Cerebellar hypoplasia
Cerebellar vermis hypoplasia
Chorea
Clonus
Congenital onset
Dystonia
Extrapyramidal dyskinesia
Feeding difficulties
Feeding difficulties in infancy
Generalized hypotonia
Gliosis
Hypoplasia of the brainstem
Hypoplasia of the corpus callosum

continues

Table 8–1. *continued*

Medical Terms
Hypoplasia of the pons
Impaired smooth pursuit
Limb hypertonia
Microcephaly
Muscular hypotonia of the trunk
Opisthotonus
Poor suck
Progressive microcephaly
Restlessness
Seizures
Severe global developmental delay
Sloping forehead
Visual impairment

Source: Adapted from "The Human Phenotype Ontology," by S. Köhler, N. A. Vasilevsky, M. Engelstad, E. Foster, J. McMurry, S. Aymé, . . . & M. Brudno (2016). The human phenotype ontology in 2017. *Nucleic Acids Research, 45*(D1), D865–D876.

Etiology

Currently, all of the identified forms of pontocerebellar hypoplasia are inherited in an autosomal recessive pattern. This means that both copies of the related gene in each cell have mutations. In other words, both parents of the individual with PCH must each carry one copy of the mutated gene, but they themselves do not have any manifested signs or symptoms of the disease. Consequently, a child inheriting two damaged copies of the gene will have PCH. According to Genetics Home Medicine (2009), mutations in the genes that produce PCH cause errors in the production of the enzymes important for the development of nerve cells, as well as for processing of ribonucleic acid (RNA): the polymeric molecule essential the expression of genes. However, the precise mechanism that causes PCH to arrest the development of the pons and cerebellum is not very well understood.

Epidemiology

PCH appears to affect both males and females equally, but the exact incidence is still generally unknown. To date, PCH subtype 2 (PCH2) is reported in at least 81 families, although more than 100 cases of different subtypes have been reported in the medical literature.

Clinical Presentation

An important manifestation of PCH2 is that the mother usually experiences an unremarkable pregnancy. Newborns tend to have no external dysmorphic features or even visceral abnormalities.

Affected infants usually present with dysphagia, largely because of the buccopharyngeal incoordination, general feeding problems, respiratory difficulties, and clonus. Extra-pyramidal dyskinesia with mixed spasticity such as **chorea**, **athetosis**, and **dystonia** appear in the later developmental stages of growth. Outcomes are very grave for infants with PCH2. The clinical symptoms of the disease become progressively worse. Children develop progressive microcephaly, central visual impairment, seizures, and impaired cognitive and motor skills. Significant in this progression of worsening symptoms are poor head control, lack of hand coordination, and absent speech and communication abilities (Namavar et al., 2011). Although, in a few cases, survival has occasionally exceeded 20 years. In the majority of cases, death is often before the age of 10 years. It is likely that improved care and tube feedings may have contributed to improved survival in some cases (Namavar, Eggens, Barth, & Baas, 2016).

Management of Dysphagia

The treatment of PCH is generally symptomatic and supportive. A multidisciplinary team approach is necessary. The team may include the pediatrician, pediatric neurologist, pediatric surgeon, speech-language pathologist, ophthalmologist, physical therapist, occupational therapist, and other disciplines the individual case may require.

The nature of dysphagia in most cases is contingent on the clinical manifestations of the infant. For example, some infants present with facial weakness and lingual weakness with fasciculations. These characteristics largely influence their ability to suck. In many of these cases, gastrostomy feeding tubes are essential for adequate nutrition.

In an extensive study of PCH2, Sánchez, Frölich, Barth, Steinlin, and Krägeloh-Mann (2014) studied 63 patients who presented with feeding difficulties, gastroesophageal reflux disease (GERD), sleep disorders, and recurrent infections. The feeding difficulties were marked by incoordination of sucking and swallowing, frequent aspiration during attempts to swallow, and taking greater than 30 min to consume meals. The feeding difficulties started in the first 6 months and subsided in only two of the 32 patients who learned to eat small amounts of mechanical soft foods. The other children tolerated small amounts of pureed foods. Twenty-two of these patients had to have a feeding tube by 3 years of age. Overall dysphagia was the predominant difficulty most of these children manifested.

Summary

As noted previously, pontocerebellar hypoplasia (PCH) is a term used to describe a rare heterogeneous group of neurodegenerative disorders with a prenatal onset. The disorder affects the ventral pons and cerebellum; two structures that share similar neuronal origins during the development of the brain. There are several subtypes of PCH, 11 have been identified at the writing of this text. PCH subtype 2 (PCH2) is the most common of these rare subtypes. PCH2 anatomically shows sparing of the spinal motor neurons and is characterized by developmental delay, language impairment, dysphagia, progressive microcephaly, and dystonia. Life expectancy rarely extends beyond puberty, although in some rare cases, individuals have survived beyond two decades. To date, there is no cure for this disease. Management tends to be supportive and symptomatic.

References

Barth, P. G. (1993). Pontocerebellar hypoplasias: An overview of a group of inherited neurodegenerative disorders with fetal onset. *Brain and Development, 15*(6), 411–422.

Barth, P. G., Vrensen, G. F. J. M., Uylings, H. B. M., Oorthuys, J. W. E., & Stam, F. C. (1990). Inherited syndrome of microcephaly, dyskinesia and pontocerebellar hypoplasia: A systemic atrophy with early onset. *Journal of the Neurological Sciences, 97*(1), 25–42.

Eggens, V. R. C. (2016). *On the origin of pontocerebellar hypoplasia: Finding genes for a rare disease.*

Genetics Home Reference. (2009). *Pontocerebellar hypoplasia.* Retrieved from https://ghr.nlm.nih.gov/condition/pontocerebellar-hypoplasia

Krause, K. (1929). IV. Nevus flammeus and glaucoma. *Ophthalmologica, 68*(4–5), 244–260.

Köhler, S., Vasilevsky, N. A., Engelstad, M., Foster, E., McMurry, J., Aymé, S., . . . & Brudno, M. (2016). The human phenotype ontology in 2017. *Nucleic Acids Research, 45*(D1), D865–D876.

Namavar, Y., Chitayat, D., Barth, P. G., Van Ruissen, F., De Wissel, M. B., Poll-The, B. T., . . . Baas, F. (2011). TSEN54 mutations cause ponto-cerebellar hypoplasia type 5. *European Journal of Human Genetics, 19*(6), 724.

Namavar, Y., Eggens, V. R., Barth, P. G., & Baas, F. (2016). *TSEN54-Related Pontocerebellar Hypoplasia*. Seattle, WA: University of Washington.

Norman, R. M., & Urich, H. (1960). The influence of a vascular factor on the distribution of symmetrical cerebral calcifications. *Journal of Neurology, Neurosurgery, and Psychiatry, 23*(2), 142.

Sánchez-Albisua, I., Frölich, S., Barth, P. G., Steinlin, M., & Krägeloh-Mann, I. (2014). Natural course of pontocerebellar hypoplasia type 2A. *Orphanet Journal of Rare Diseases, 9*(1), 70.

van Dijk, T., Baas, F., Barth, P. G., & Poll-The, B.T. (2018). What's new in pontocerebellar hypoplasia? An update on genes and subtypes. *Orphanet Journal of Rare Diseases, 13*(1), 92.

9

Fahr's Disease

KEY WORDS: encephalopathy, Fahr's disease, thalamus, hippocampus, calcification, ossification, pigmentary retinopathy

Definition

Fahr's disease (FD) is a rare, genetically dominant neurological disorder. It is characterized by abnormal deposits of calcium in areas of the brain that are essential for movement such as the basal ganglia, **thalamus**, **hippocampus**, cerebral cortex cerebellar, subcortical white matter, and dentate nucleus. The disorder is manifested in an array of symptoms such as progressive deterioration of motor function, declining intellect, seizures, motor speech disorders, spasticity, visual impairments, dysphagia, dystonia, psychiatric disturbances, and parkinsonism. The Parkinson-like symptoms usually evolve later in the progression of the disease. Generally, Fahr's syndrome is considered a combination of **encephalopathy** and progressive calcification of the basal ganglia. Diagnosis is established mainly by brain imaging, even though lab tests are needed to exclude other causes of brain calcification (Lima & Rodrigues, 2017).

The onset of Fahr's is typically around the fourth or fifth decade of life, but it occasionally occurs in childhood as well as in adolescence. There does not appear to be a correlation between age, the amount of **calcification** that occurs in the brain, and the neurological deficit. Since calcification is age dependent, it is unlikely that it would be present in individuals under 50 years of age (National Institute of Neurological Disorders and Stroke, 2019).

History

The German neurologist Theodore Fahr is often credited as the first person to identify the disease that now bears his name. Back in 1930, he described an 81-year-old patient with dementia and "immobility without paralysis." However, it was Delacour in 1850 who was the first to recognize "**ossification** of brain capillaries" in a 56-year-old male patient whom he described as having immobility and stiffness of the lower extremities with accompanying tremors (Batla & Tai, 2015). Later, Bamberger (1855) described a female with intellectual challenges and seizures with cerebral vessel calcifications. However, Fahr's description was considered the first to identify and label idiopathic non-arteriosclerotic cerebral calcification. Boller, Boller, and Gilbert (1977) shed more light on the disease when they described nine members of the same family with familial idiopathic brain calcification (Batla & Tai, 2015).

Etiology

Although FD is associated with a variety of medical conditions, the exact etiology remains unclear. Some conditions appear to be endocrine disorders, mitochondrial myopathies, dermatological disorders, or infectious diseases (Saleem et al., 2013). Movement disorders are the most typical manifestation of Fahr's disease, and Parkinsonism accounts for 57% (Otu, Anikwe, & Cocker,

2015). However, it is generally accepted that Fahr's is familial and inherited. Autosomal dominant cases make up 60% of diagnoses (Ashtari & Fatehi 2010). Calcification of the basal ganglia, which is the main disturbance in Fahr's, can occur with infectious, metabolic, as well as genetic disorders (Fenichel, 2009).

If the etiology is endocrine, then parathyroid disturbances tend to be most prominent. According to Saleem et al. (2013), hypothyroidism may also be associated with disorders such as dysarthria, cataract, seizures, congestive heart failure, dental dysplasia, and dental cavities.

Fahr's disease usually has its onset in adulthood with a manifestation of neurodegenerative conditions. As a neurodegeneration with brain iron accumulation disease (NBIA), it presents with progressive dystonia, basal ganglia calcification dysarthria, along with rigidity and **pigmentary retinopathy** (Saleem et al., 2013). In addition, adult onset chorea and mild cognitive dysfunction have been present in the disorder. See Table 9–1 for some of the etiological presentations of Fahr's disease.

Table 9–1. Etiological Manifestations of Fahr's Syndrome

Condition	Manifested Symptoms
Endocrine Disorders	Hypothyroidism: dysarthria, dysphagia, seizures, dental dysplasia, dental caries, congestive heart failure, anemia
Adult-Onset Neurodegenerative Conditions	Dystonia, impaired cognition, dementia, rigidity, pigmentary retinopathy
Dermatological Disorders	Seizures, dementia, skin and mucous membrane disorders
Infectious Diseases	Rubella, herpes, cytomegalovirus (CMV), Cockayne syndrome types 1 & 2
Inherited or Early-Onset Syndromes	Aicardi-Gouteres syndrome, tuberous sclerosis complex, brucellosis, Coats' disease

It is important to bear in mind that within FD there are several factors such as inherited disorders, radiation, chemotherapy, as well as carbon monoxide poisoning that can contribute to brain calcification. Additionally, the manifestation of FD as well as the outcomes can differ from person to person. One fact that appears to be clear is that FD is progressive and no known cure has been identified.

Epidemiology

The true prevalence of FD is relatively unknown. It may occur in a sporadic or a familial fashion. It is believed to have autosomal dominant inheritance, but some cases may have autosomal recessive inheritance. Its prevalence is reportedly to be less than 1 in 1,000,000. Only a handful of cases have been reported in the literature, and of those that are documented, there is a higher reported incidence among males compared to females. Onset is typically around the third to sixth decade of life. In addition, two peaks of maximum occurrence have been identified in the literature. At the beginning of the adult-stage onset of the disorder, patients tend to manifest more psychiatric disorders; whereas in the later years, such as 50 to 60, symptomatology tends to be cognitive and psychomotor changes.

Clinical Presentation

The diagnosis of Fahr's disease is usually determined when other conditions that may also cause bilateral calcification of the basal ganglia and other brain regions are ruled out. Typically, radiographic imaging of the brain will show the presence of whitish concentrated radiopaque regions in the most involved areas, such as the basal ganglia (Bekiesinska-Figatowska, Mierzewska, & Jurkiewicz, 2013).

Table 9–2. Clinical Features of Fahr's Disease

Category	Clinical Features
Neurological	Seizures, spasticity, dysarthria, dementia, myoclonus intracranial hypertension, dystonia, loss of consciousness, speech disorders (dysarthria), swallowing problems, paroxysmal choreothetosis
Movement Disorders	Clumsiness, fatigability, gait disorders, myoclonus, muscle cramps
Neuropsychiatric	Psychoses, depression, intellectual decline, decreased organizational skills

Source: Adapted from "Fahr's Syndrome: Literature Review of Current Evidence," by S. Saleem, H. M. Aslam, M. Anwar, S. Anwar, M. Saleem, A. Saleem, and M. A. K. Rehmani, 2013, *Orphanet Journal of Rare Diseases, 8*(1), 156.

Since there are myriad conditions that produce intracerebral as well as basal ganglia calcifications, Fahr's disease must be diagnosed based on clinical and neurological findings as well as the exclusion of other primary causes (Gligorievski, 2018).

A variety of neurological signs and symptoms are associated with Fahr's disease. Some of these are clumsiness, persistent fatigue, gait disorder, speech deficits, dementia, Parkinsonism, epilepsy, chorea, dystonia, and tics (Table 9–2). The main neurological manifestations of Fahr's disease include motor disorders such as Parkinsonism, dystonia, tics, dysarthria, and epilepsy. It is important to note that either one of these manifestations can produce the dysphagia typically seen in Fahr's. So, while the diagnosis of Fahr's disease may not actually cause dysphagia, the manifested symptoms such as the dystonia, parkinsonism, and even the dysarthria, for example, may very well be contributing factors. For example, dysarthria is the name given to a family of motor speech disorders that in all cases involve weakness, slowness, and/or lack of coordination of the speech musculature because of damage to the central or peripheral nervous system (Yorkston & Beukelman, 2004). As it turns out, most of the muscles involved in speech are also engaged in the swallowing process, particularly at the oral phase of swallowing. In fact, Lima and Rodrigues (2017) reported dysphagia as the initial symptom in a patient with Fahr's disease.

Clinical Manifestations

There have been accounts on the literature regarding changes in the orofacial motor functions of individuals with Fahr's disease. Patients with Fahr's disease show difficulty in coordination of the speech musculature, which ultimately interferes with swallowing skills. Santos, Fraga, and Cardoso (2014) reported a case in which a patient with Fahr's disease presented with poor lip seal resulting in drooling, reduced posterior propulsion of the bolus, and multiple swallows to clear bolus. The general findings for this patient were oropharyngeal dysphagia, characterized by decreased oral control and pharyngolaryngeal dysmotility.

The manifestations of dysphagia in Fahr's disease differ based on the symptomatology and severity of the disease. For example, individuals with Fahr's who manifest significant muscle weakness may have difficulty masticating and forming the bolus; they may also have difficulty in posterior bolus propulsion. Even though treatment here may be on a case-by-case presentation, there is still the general rule of clinical and instrumental assessment to determine the precise nature of the problem and to administer the appropriate type of food texture or liquid consistency based on the findings. Both patient and family may require education or reeducation regarding diet safety.

In their longitudinal study of swallowing in Fahr's disease, Griesemer, Lasker, Nimmons, Hastings, Petrof, West, and Griesemer (2007) found that as motoric skills declined, the patient exhibited severe oral stage impairments characterized by decreased lingual movement that resulted in delayed swallow at the oral stage. In terms of the pharyngeal stage, difficulty occurred with liquids, and solids adhered to the pyriforms and to the pharyngeal walls. Obviously, because of the rarity of the disease, reports of the characteristics of dysphagia in Fahr's disease are only as per case. Nevertheless, the picture that emerges from the few cases is one that depicts dysphagia resulting from the reduced motor movement present in the disorder. This is manifested in deficits in the musculature integral for mastication and bolus propulsion, resulting in the type of oral pharyngeal dysphagia described.

Management of Dysphagia

There is currently no cure for Fahr's disease, nor is there a standard regimen of treatment. Treatment is directed toward controlling the manifested symptoms of the disease. In the case of dysphagia in Fahr's, treatment is determined by the presenting dysphagic symptoms. The management of dysphagia in this disease is largely based upon (1) the presenting symptoms, (2) the type, and (3) the severity of the dysphagia. Once the presence of a swallowing problem has been identified, the speech-language pathologist will make a determination as to the appropriate treatment protocol. Some of the treatments may involve adjusting the food textures and viscosity of liquids, utilizing postural adjustments, as well as specific techniques. In some severe cases in which the patient is at perpetual risk of aspiration pneumonia, alternative feeding such as a gastrostomy feeding tube may be considered.

Summary

Fahr's disease is a rare, neurological disorder that has an autosomal dominant pattern. It is linked to a variety of other diseases, but no single etiologic agent has been currently identified. It is characterized by abnormal deposits of calcium in areas of the brain that are all essential for movement such as the basal ganglia, thalamus, hippocampus, cerebral cortex cerebellar, subcortical white matter, and dentate nucleus. The onset of Fahr's is typically around the fourth or fifth decade of life, but it occasionally occurs in childhood as well as in adolescence. Since there are myriad conditions that produce intracerebral as well as basal ganglia calcifications, Fahr's disease is generally diagnosed based on clinical and neurological findings as well as the exclusion of other primary causes. To date, there is still no known cure for Fahr's, but treatment is based on the manifested symptoms.

References

Ashtari, F., & Fatehi, F. (2010). Fahr's disease: Variable presentations in a family. *Neurological Sciences, 31*(5), 66–67.

Bamberger, P. H. (1855). Beobactungen und bemerkungen uber hirnkrankheiten. *Verhandlungen Physikalisch-Medizinische Gesellschaft Würzburg, 6,* 325–328.

Batla, A., & Tai, X. Y. (2015). Fahr's disease: Current perspectives. *Dovepress Open Access, 2015,* 43–49. doi: https://doi.org/10.2147/ODRR .S63388

Bekiesinska-Figatowska, M., Mierzewska, H., & Jurkiewicz, E. (2013). Basal ganglia lesions in children and adults. *European Journal of Radiology, 82*(5), 837–849.

Boller, F., Boller, M., & Gilbert, J. (1977). Familial idiopathic cerebral calcifications. *Journal of Neurology, Neurosurgery & Psychiatry, 40*(3), 280–285.

Fenichel, G. M. (2009). *Clinical pediatric neurology: A signs and symptoms approach.* Philadelphia, AP: Elsevier Health Sciences.

Gligorievski, A. (2018). U.S. diagnosis of acute appendicitis. *Medcrave Online Journal Anatomy & Physiology, 5*(3), 225–229.

Griesemer, J., Lasker, J. P., Nimmons, E., Hastings, J., Petrof, R., & West J. (2007, November). *Longitudinal changes in communication, cognition, and swallowing in Fahr's disease.* Paper presented at the Technical Session at the ASHA Convention, Boston, MA.

Hanson, E. K., Yorkston, K. M., & Beukelman, D. R. (2004). Speech supplementation techniques for dysarthria: A systematic review. In *Data-*

base of *Abstracts of Reviews of Effects (DARE): Quality-assessed reviews [Internet].* York, UK: Centre for Reviews and Dissemination.

Lima, J., & Rodrigues, B. (2017). Dysphagia in a patient with Fahr's disease. *Neurology, 18*(16 Suppl.), P2.212.

National Institute of Neurological Disorders and Stroke. (2019). Fahr's Syndrome Information Page. Retrieved 10 June 2019 from https:// www.ninds.nih.gov/Disorders/All-Disorders/Fahrs-Syndrome -Information-Page

Otu, A. A., Anikwe, J. C., & Cocker, D. (2015). Fahr's disease: A rare neurological presentation in a tropical setting. *Clinical Case Reports, 3*(10), 806.

Saleem, S., Aslam, H. M., Anwar, M., Anwar, S., Saleem, M., Saleem, A., & Rehmani, M. A. K. (2013). Fahr's syndrome: Literature review of current evidence. *Orphanet Journal of Rare Diseases, 8*(1), 156.

Santos, K. W. D., Fraga, B. F. D., & Cardoso, M. C. D. A. F. (2014). Dysfunctions of the stomatognathic system and vocal aspects in Fahr disease: Case report. *CoDAS, 26*(2), 164–167.

Yorkston, K. M., & Beukelman, D. R. (2004). Dysarthria: Tools for clinical decision-making. *The ASHA Leader, 9*(9), 4–21.

10

Biotin-Thiamine-Responsive Basal Ganglia Disease

KEY WORDS: biotin-thiamine, dystonia

Definition

Biotin-thiamine-responsive basal ganglia disease (BTBGD), also known as biotin-responsive basal ganglia disease (BBGD), is a rare, autosomal recessive neurometabolic disorder. It is caused by a defect in the gene that provides the instructions needed for the thiamine transporter protein to carry the vitamin thiamine (Kono et al., 2009). This vitamin is obtained from foods and carried into the cells. The age of onset varies, but the disorder commonly occurs between 3 and 4 years of age. As its name suggests, the main area affected in the brain is the basal ganglia, which is important for the control of movement. The severity of the disease as well as the associated signs and symptoms vary from person to person. BTBGD is characterized by subacute encephalopathy, confusion, seizure, dysarthria, dysphagia, and **dystonia**. If untreated with biotin and thiamine, it is usually fatal.

115

History

BTBGD was first described in 1998 by Ozand et al., who classified the disorder as biotin-responsive basal ganglia disease. Then in 2013, the disorder was renamed by Alfadhel et al. as biotin-thiamine-responsive basal ganglia disease. Ozand et al. found the disorder in 10 patients: 8 of whom were from Saudi Arabia, 1 from Syria, and the other from Yemen. Subsequently, cases were reported in other ethnic groups such as Lebanese, Portuguese, East Indian, and Japanese, but these were mostly small numbers. To date, fewer than 40 cases have been reported worldwide.

Etiology

Biotin-thiamine-responsive basal ganglia disease is caused by mutations in the SLC19A3 gene. This gene provides instructions for making a protein called thiamine transporter, which moves a vitamin called thiamine into the cells. Thiamine, also recognized as vitamin B1, is obtained from food. BTBGD is inherited in an autosomal recessive manner. This means both copies of the gene in each cell will have mutations. The parents of an individual with an autosomal recessive condition each carry one copy of the mutated gene. Mutations in the SLC19A3 gene appear to result in a protein that is incapable of transporting thiamine into the cells, thus leading to decreased absorption of the vitamin, resulting in neurological dysfunction. The lesions produced by the disorder are seen throughout the brain, most notably in the basal ganglia.

Epidemiology

The prevalence of BTBGD is still largely unknown. So far, just a few cases have been reported in the medical literature, and most of these were from Arab populations (Genetics Home Reference, 2019). BTBGD is common in children, especially those between 3 to 10 years of age, although there has been at least one report of the disorder in a 30-day-old baby (Perez-Duenas et al., 2013) and another report of the disorder in a 20-year-old individual (Debs et al., 2010).

Clinical Presentation

Some reports have recognized BTBGD to occur in three stages: stage 1—subacute encephalopathy, which usually presents with a fever as the first warning sign and accompanying confusion; stage 2—acute encephalopathy with accompanying seizures, dysphagia, and motor speech deficits; and stage 3—a chronic or slowly progressive encephalopathy that has the potential to lead to death. Each stage has its own unique set of symptoms, as displayed in Table 10–1 (Aljabri, Kamal, Arif, Al Qaedi, &

Table 10–1. Clinical Stages of Biotin-Thiamine-Responsive Basal Ganglia Disease

Stage	Disease Characteristics
Stage 1: Subacute encephalopathy	Fever, emesis, and confusion
Stage 2: Acute encephalopathy	Seizures, quadriparesis or quadriplegia, loss of developmental milestones, dysphagia, and dysarthria
Stage 3: Chronic or slowly progressive encephalopath	Akinetic mute state, permanent loss of speech and auditory comprehension, and imminent death

Source: Adapted from "A Case Report of Biotin-Thiamine-Responsive Basal Ganglia Disease in a Saudi Child: Is Extended Genetic Family Study Recommended?" by M. F. Aljabri, N. M. Kamal, M. Arif, A. M. Al Qaedi, and E. Y. Santali, 2016, *Medicine, 95*(40).

Santali, 2016; Ozand et al., 1998). Generally, in the case of sub-acute encephalopathy, the manifested symptoms are confusion, seizures, ataxia, dystonia, supranuclear facial palsy, ophthalmo-plegia, and dysphagia. If left untreated, these symptoms can eventually prove fatal. In some cases, BTBGD presents insidiously, with slow progression of the symptoms discussed previously in this section. Even though the disease is rare, an encouraging factor is that prompt administration of biotin and thiamine early in the detection of the disease can result in partial or complete improvement within days (Tabarki, Al-Hashem, & Alfadhel, 2013).

Management of Dysphasia

There is no cure for BTBGD because it is a genetic condition. However, treatment focuses on managing the symptoms of the disorder. Nevertheless, treatment with the vitamins biotin and thiamine are relatively successful in managing the symptoms. Some of the major complications of BTBGD are swallowing and speech difficulty.

The nature of the dysphagia in BTBGD has not been very well described in the literature. For example, Debs et al. (2010) described the presence of "swallowing dysfunction" amidst an array of other deficits such as loss of speech, confusion, and seizures in two European cases of BTBGD. Once the patients were administered the biotin or combination of biotin and thiamine early in the disease course, the symptoms that identified the condition were alleviated. Ozand et al. (1998) described a similar set of circumstances in 10 patients diagnosed with BTBGD. These authors claimed that the symptoms of BTBGD, including dysphagia, were reversed following the **biotin-thiamine** treatment.

In the majority of cases, early detection of the disease as well as early administration of the drug treatment is essential to the management of dysphagia in this disease. To date, only a small number of cases of BTBGD have been reported in the medical literature and, furthermore, the extent and type of dysphagia is largely unknown.

Summary

Biotin-thiamine-responsive basal ganglia disease is a rare disorder that affects the nervous system, including the basal ganglia that is integral for the control of movement. The disease for the most part tends to affect individuals from Arab populations. The symptoms of the disease are usually manifested between the ages of 3 to 10 years, although the disorder has appeared both much earlier and much later in a few cases. Most of the neurological problems affect movement. The movement problems in turn affect the facial muscles, leading to difficulty chewing and swallowing. There is no cure for BTBGD, but the symptoms are managed completely or partially by biotin and thiamine medications that must be maintained for life.

References

Alfadhel, M., Almuntashri, M., Jadah, R. H., Bashiri, F. A., Al Rifai, M. T., Al Shalaan, H., . . . & Al-Twaijri, W. (2013). Biotin-responsive basal ganglia disease should be renamed biotin-thiamine-responsive basal ganglia disease: A retrospective review of the clinical, radiological and molecular findings of 18 new cases. *Orphanet Journal of Rare Diseases, 8*(1), 83.

Aljabri, M. F., Kamal, N. M., Arif, M., Al Qaedi, A. M., & Santali, E. Y. (2016). A case report of biotin-thiamine-responsive basal ganglia disease in a Saudi child: Is extended genetic family study recommended? *Medicine, 95*(40).

Debs, R., Depienne, C., Rastetter, A., Bellanger, A., Degos, B., Galanaud, D., . . . Sedel, F. (2010). Biotin-responsive basal ganglia disease in ethnic Europeans with novel SLC19A3 mutations. *Archives of Neurology, 67*(1), 126–130.

Genetics Home Reference. (2019). Biotin-thiamine-responsive basal ganglia disease. Retrieved from https://ghr.nlm.nih.gov/condition /biotin-thiamine-responsive-basal-ganglia-disease

Kono, S., Miyajima, H., Yoshida, K., Togawa, A., Shirakawa, K., & Suzuki, H. (2009). Mutations in a thiamine-transporter gene and Wernicke-like encephalopathy. *New England Journal of Medicine, 360*(17), 1792–1794.

Ozand, P. T., Gascon, G. G., Al Essa, M., Joshi, S., Al Jishi, E., Bakheet, S., . . . Dabbagh, O. (1998). Biotin-responsive basal ganglia disease: A novel entity. *Brain: A Journal of Neurology, 121*(7), 1267–1279.

Pérez-Dueñas, B., Serrano, M., Rebollo, M., Muchart, J., Gargallo, E., Dupuits, C., & Artuch, R. (2013). Reversible lactic acidosis in a newborn with thiamine transporter-2 deficiency. *Pediatrics, 131*(5), e1670–e1675.

Tabarki, B., Al-Hashem, A., & Alfadhel, M. (2013). Biotin-thiamine-responsive basal ganglia disease. In *GeneReviews®[Internet]*. Seattle, WA: University of Washington.

11

Pompe Disease

KEY WORDS: Pompe disease, acid alpha-glucosidase (GAA), glycogen

Definition

Pompe disease (PD) is inherited as an autosomal recessive genetic trait. It is a rare and often fatal disease. The disorder is caused by the buildup of a complex sugar called **glycogen** in the cells of the body. This buildup is due to pathogenic variations in the gene that carries the information for the production and function of a protein called **acid alpha-glucosidase** (GAA). A shortage of this protein or enzyme will prevent glycogen in the cells from breaking down to a simple sugar such as glucose. Failure to break down the glycogen will result in the accumulation of glycogen in the body's tissue, particularly in the skeletal muscles—smooth as well as cardiac muscles. Glycogen is an important energy source found in most tissues, but it is especially abundant in the liver and in the muscles. In the liver, it serves as a glucose reserve for the maintenance of normoglycemia; whereas in the muscles, the glycogen provides energy for muscle contraction. Thus, PD is one of the diseases known as lysosomal storage disorders (LSDs).

Other synonyms for this disorder are glycogen storage disease type II, acid maltase deficiency (AMD), and acid alpha-glucosidase (GAA) deficiency.

All patients with Pompe disease share the same disease course, such as progressive debilitation, organ failure, and even death. The first symptoms of PD can occur at any age from birth to late adulthood. However, there are some clinical differences based on time of onset. Earlier onset of the disease is usually associated with greater severity and more rapid progression of the disease, compared to later onset (National Organization for Rare Disorders, 2019). Infants who are severely affected usually manifest symptoms during the first 3 months after birth. The enlargement of the heart is the primary deficit at this early stage of life. Severity varies not only based on age of onset, but also on the particular organ involved, the degree of muscular involvement, and the rate of progression (Kishnani et al., 2006). Kisnani et al. classified PD as infantile and late onset—also referred to as juvenile/adult. Each group presents with unique symptoms of the disorder. Generally, the infantile onset is distinguished by the rapidity of the symptoms, most notably the hypertrophic cardiomyopathy. On the other hand, the juvenile/adult onset presents with the primary symptom of muscle weakness, which then progresses to respiratory problems that may prove fatal.

History

Pompe disease has a rather interesting history. It is the eponym of Johann Pompe, a Dutch physician who first discovered the disease in 1932. He described the disease in a 7-month-old infant who presented with cardiac problems and generalized muscle weakness. Critical to Dr. Pompe's observation was the fact that the infant exhibited vacuolar glycogen storage in tissues throughout the body. Following his discovery, similar cases were also reported (Lim, Li, & Raben, 2014). Cori (1954) classified the disease as glycogen storage disease type II because of the abnormal metabolism of glycogen. However, shortly after, Hers (1963) discovered an enzyme called maltase that proved to be critical to the breakdown of glycogen to glucose. Furthermore, Hers discovered that this enzyme is not only found in the lysosomes, but it is the single glycogen-degrading enzyme present in the lysosomes. Based on this seminal work by Hers, the concept of lysosomal storage diseases was established (Lim et al., 2014). Hers' research definitively connected the link between the enzyme maltase and glycogen. Thus, Pompe's seminal discovery almost three decades prior established the disease that now bears his name.

Etiology

PD is a genetic condition. It is associated with pathogenic differences in the acid alpha-glucosidase (GAA) gene. So far, approximately 500 variations of the GAA gene have been identified in individuals with the disorder. It is inherited in an autosomal recessive pattern. Recessive genetic disorders occur when an individual inherits two copies of an altered gene for the same trait, one from each parent. This means that if an individual inherits one normal gene and one altered gene, that person would be a carrier for the disease, but will not typically exhibit symptoms of the disease. The risk for two carrier parents to both pass on the altered gene and have a child with the disorder is 25% with each pregnancy, but the risk to have a child who is a carrier like the parents increases to 50%. On the other hand, the chances of a child receiving normal genes from both parents remains 25%. There is no gender difference in this inheritance pattern.

The first signs and symptoms of PD can occur at any age from birth to late adulthood. The timing of the onset is associated, for the most part, with the severity of the pathogenic variations in each of the two GAA gene copies in the patient (Hagemans et al., 2005).

Epidemiology

PD occurs in various populations and ethnic groups worldwide. Estimates may vary, but the incidence in the United States of all forms of PD is around 1 in 40,000 births. The disease affects males and females equally. Unfortunately, not all individuals with PD are readily diagnosed. According to reports from the National Organization for Rare diseases (2019), in the past few years, several cases of PD have been identified among individuals with limb-girdle dystrophies and/or high levels of creatine kinase in the blood. Dutch studies report an estimated frequency of the late onset form of PD to be 1 in 57,000 (Ausems et al., 1999). However, as is the case with rare diseases, it is difficult to be exact about how many individuals are truly affected. From the assumed data, it is estimated that the current worldwide prevalence is probably about 5,000 to 10,000 persons with the disease (Ausems et al., 1999). Nevertheless, incidence data are difficult to fully ascertain since reports in the literature range from 1 in 14,000 to 1 in 300,000, all heavily dependent on ethnicity and geographical location (Hirschhorn & Reuser, 2001).

Many studies suggest that the incidence of PD may very well vary across ethnicities. Hirschhorn and Reuser report that Pompe disease is more common among African American and Chinese infants, while the juvenile/adult form of Pompe appears to be higher among the Dutch population (Ausems et al., 1999). See Table 11–1 for PD across various ethnic groups and populations.

Clinical Presentation

Pompe disease has a heterogeneous clinical presentation as well as diverse rates of progression (Table 11–2). The infantile onset form usually appears within the first few months of life. This form is typically multisystem and tends to progress rapidly with severe cardiomyopathy and respiratory failure, and is usually

Table 11–1. Incidence of Pompe Disease Across Various Ethnic Groups and Populations

Ethnic Group/ Population	Incidence	Source
African American	1 per 14,000 infantile onset 1 per 40,000 including all forms	Hirschhorn & Reuser (2001)
Netherlands	1 per 138,000 infantile onset 1 per 57,000 juvenile/adult onset	Ausems et al. (1999)
United States	1 per 40,000 including all forms	Martiniuk, Chen, & Mack (1998)
China	1 per 50,000 all forms	Lin, Hwang, Hsiao, & Jin (1987)
European Descent	1 per 100,000 infantile onset 1 per 60,000 juvenile/adult onset	Martiniuk, Chen, & Mack (1998)
Australia	1 per 145,000 all forms	Meikle et al. (1999)
Portugal	1 per 600,00 all forms	Pinto et al. (2004)

fatal within the first year of life. Patients with this classic infantile PD are the most severely affected. Hardly any symptoms are apparent at birth, but the disease tends to appear within the first three months of life with rapidly progressive muscle weakness (known as "floppy infants"), diminished muscle tone, and respiratory problems. On the other hand, the diagnosis of PD in the juvenile/adult form can be more challenging as these patients generally present with a slower progression of symptoms. In this group, the onset of the disease is most often dominated by skeletal muscle weakness affecting proximal limb-girdle and respiratory musculature (Dasouki et al. 2014; Lukacs et al., 2016; Marsden, 2005).

Furthermore, in the juvenile/adult onset of PD, the range of clinical presentation can vary from asymptomatic patients to

Table 11–2. Clinical Symptoms of Pompe Disease

Infantile Onset Symptoms (4–8 months)	Juvenile/Adult Onset Symptoms (>1 year–adulthood)
Weakness in the arms and legs	Muscle weakness (legs, trunk, arms)
Hypotonia	Rigid spine syndrome
Hepatomegaly	Muscle cramps
Respiratory difficulties	Walking difficulties
Cardiomyopathy (often severe)	Respiratory difficulties (diaphragm and accessory muscles)
Feeding problems	
Macroglossia	Difficulty swallowing
Failure to thrive	Weight loss
Hearing loss	(Disease progression varies, but is slower than in infantile onset; age of death varies from childhood to adulthood and is due to respiratory failure)
(Rapid disease progression; death in the first year of life due to cardio–respiratory failure or pneumonia)	

severe proximal and diaphragmatic myopathy with a need for ventilation support (Güngör et al., 2013). It is well reported in the literature that feeding and swallowing difficulties are common in infantile PD. However, there are studies that have also reported significant swallowing deficits in patients with late onset PD. Maggi et al. (2013) described three family members with late onset PD characterized by brain stem symptoms who presented, most notably, with swallowing difficulty and tongue weakness. One patient in this study had difficulty moving the lips as well as facial weakness. Typically, tongue weakness with macroglossia (the abnormal enlargement of the tongue) is more common in early onset PD. However, Dubrovsky, Corderi, Lin, Kishnani, and Jones (2011) reported that of the19 patients affected with PD in their study, one-third of them exhibited swallowing problems, particularly difficulty manipulating the bolus due to lingual weakness.

Dysphagia in PD

Dubrovsky et al. (2011) noted that the root cause of the dysphagia in their patients was tongue hypotrophy. In another study, Hobson-Webb, Jones, and Kishnani (2013) reported that their patients with late onset PD exhibited oropharyngeal dysphagia—again characterized by tongue weakness. It would appear that tongue weakness associated with dysphagia might be a more frequent part of the clinical picture in late onset PD than hitherto reported. Jones, Crisp, Asrani, Sloane, and Kishnani (2014) reported that 71% of their patients with late onset Pompe disease exhibited lingual weakness. Their study suggests that lingual strength assessment might be an important factor in the differential diagnosis of late onset PD. Furthermore, this deficit most likely accounts for the oropharyngeal dysphagia that now appears to be present in late onset Pompe disease.

Feeding and swallowing difficulties have been consistently reported and have now become part of the PD phenotype, but the characterization of the dysphagia is only now emerging. Fecarotta et al. (2013) observed that the pathophysiology of dysphagia in PD patients is not as clearly defined as in other disorders, such as strokes. However, in PD, it is speculated that different mechanisms may coalesce to cause an abnormal swallowing disorder. For example, the dysfunction of the bulbar muscles along with the weakness of the respiratory muscles and the diaphragm can interfere with the smooth coordination of swallowing and breathing. The study by Jones et al. (2010) identified oropharyngeal dysphagia in 13 infants with PD, most notably in one 15-day-old infant. The oral stage signs were manifested in a weak sucking pattern in approximately 77% of these patients. Pharyngeal stage problems were present in 100% of these subjects. The pharyngeal symptoms were characterized by delayed initiation of the swallow in 92% of the subjects and pharyngeal residue in 77% of the subjects. In addition, penetration and aspiration were present in about 38.4% of these patients. This study suggests that in PD, as in the more common etiologies of dysphagia, swallowing problems can occur in most stages of the swallow, particularly at the oropharyngeal stage. In fact, most of the studies of Pompe disease seem to agree that the oropharyngeal stage dysphagia is a more common occurrence in the infantile onset form of the disease, even though it is present in the adult onset form.

Management of Dysphasia

There is no cure for Pompe disease; therefore, treatment is disease specific, symptomatic, and supportive. Treatment requires the coordinative efforts of a multidisciplinary team of specialists such as neurologists, pediatricians, cardiologists, orthopedists, speech-language pathologists, physical therapists, and occupational therapists.

Enzyme Replacement Therapy (ERT)

There is significant promise in enzyme replacement therapy (ERT) with alglucosidase alfa. This drug, delivered as an infusion, is chemically an analog of the enzyme that is deficient in individuals with PD. The U.S. Food and Drug Administration (FDA) first approved this drug in 2006 for all patients with Pompe disease (Chien, Hwu, & Lee, 2013).

Studies have demonstrated that ERT significantly lengthens survival and improves motor development and cardiac function in the infant onset PD (Chien et al., 2013). Fecarotta et al. (2013) were among the first to report an in-depth assessment of the effects of ERT on dysphagia in a child with PD. This study assessed dysphagia via videofluoroscopy before the start of ERT and after 3 years of administering the therapy. Initially, the child exhibited chewing and swallowing difficulties following the diagnosis of PD around 2 years of age. At the age of 6.3 years, after 36 months of ERT, feeding difficulties were improved and no further problems with eating and drinking occurred. Subsequent studies reported improvement in some patients treated with ERT (Jones et al., 2010). However, some patients required additional speech therapy in addition to the ERT.

It is well established that PD is manifested across a broad severity spectrum; thus, it is not surprising that it responds variably to therapy. ERT has resulted in disease course stabilization with motor and pulmonary improvements. However, many factors significantly affect the outcome of treatment. Some of these factors include age at the initiation of ERT, muscle type, underlying genotype, and the multidisciplinary approach to treatment (Kishnani & Beckemeyer, 2014). Other studies have shown that patients with advance stage PD may not show much benefit from ERT; consequently, there is not much improvement in swallowing. In these cases, the purpose of ERT is usually to help the patient retain their extant level of function. Infantile PD is the most severe form. It has historically resulted in early mortality secondary to cardiopulmonary problems, but management with ERT has significantly extended the life span of most individuals in this population.

Supportive Management

Apart from ERT as a direct treatment for PD, there are other supportive and symptomatic interventions. Most patients with PD will require respiratory support because of respiration difficulties. Thus, some patients will need respiratory aid through mechanical ventilation. They may also need physical therapy and occupational therapy to improve strength and to use assistive devices.

PD weakens the muscles for mastication and deglutition. Frequently, the skills of the speech-language pathologist are required to provide support for safe swallowing. Food consistencies may have to be adjusted to facilitate ease in swallowing. Sometimes the patient and/or caregiver may have to be instructed in utilizing postural techniques and exercises in order to decrease the risk of aspiration. In some cases of infantile onset PD, if the swallowing problem becomes so severe that oral feeding is no longer an option, then alternative feeding such as a nasogastric feeding tube (NG) or a percutaneous endoscopic gastrostomy

(PEG) may be required. Some individuals with juvenile/adult onset PD may only require a soft or pureed diet to facilitate easier mastication, but few require feeding tubes.

Summary

PD is a rare, multisystem, progressive metabolic myopathy caused by pathogenic deficiency in the acid alpha-glucosidase (GAA) gene. GAA is an enzyme needed for the degradation of lysosomal glycogen. Because of the shortage of this enzyme, a complex sugar called glycogen cannot be broken down into a simple sugar such as glucose. This causes the glycogen to accumulate in virtually all muscle tissue of the body, but most notably in the skeletal muscle—smooth muscle and cardiac muscle. This accumulation of glycogen causes progressive damage to tissue structure and function. Different clinical subtypes of PD are recognized. The first subtype is severe infantile onset, which is usually manifested within the first 3 months after birth. These patients usually have enlargement of the heart in addition to widespread skeletal muscle weakness, as well as a life expectancy of less than two years if untreated. The second subtype is a more slowly progressive late onset form that occurs in children and adults. In this late onset subtype, there is a gradual manifestation of walking disability and reduced respiratory function. Most individuals with PD present with feeding problems and dysphagia, most notably oropharyngeal type. Patients are usually managed by diet modification, postural techniques, and—wherever possible—exercises. In the more severe cases of dysphagia, some patients may have to be fed via feeding tubes. While there is no cure for PD, there have been promising results in many cases with the use of enzyme replacement therapy (ERT). Studies have demonstrated that ERT significantly lengthens survival and improves motor development and cardiac function in the infant onset PD. There is some evidence to support the finding that feeding difficulties improved and no further problems with eating and drinking occurred in some patients treated with ERT.

References

Ausems, M. G. E. M., Verbiest, J., Hermans, M. M. P., Kroos, M. A., Beemer, F. A., Wokke, J. H. J., Van der Ploeg, A. T. (1999). Frequency of glycogen storage disease type II in the Netherlands: Implications for diagnosis and genetic counselling. *European Journal of Human Genetics, 7*(6), 713.

Chien, Y. H., Hwu, W. L., & Lee, N. C. (2013). Pompe disease: Early diagnosis and early treatment make a difference. *Pediatrics & Neonatology, 54*(4), 219–227.

Cori, G. T., & Schulman, J. L. (1954). Glycogen storage disease of the liver: II. Enzymic studies. *Pediatrics, 14*(6), 646–650.

Dasouki, M., Jawdat, O., Almadhoun, O., Pasnoor, M., McVey, A. L., Abuzinadah, A., . . . Dimachkie, M. M. (2014). Pompe disease: Literature review and case series. *Neurologic Clinics, 32*(3), 751–776.

Dubrovsky, A., Corderi, J., Lin, M., Kishnani, P. S., & Jones, H. N. (2011). Expanding the phenotype of late-onset pompe disease: Tongue weakness: A new clinical observation. *Muscle & Nerve, 44*(6), 897–901.

Fecarotta, S., Ascione, S., Montefusco, G., Della Casa, R., Villari, P., Romano, A., . . . Parenti, G. (2013). Improvement of dysphagia in a child affected by Pompe disease treated with enzyme replacement therapy. *Italian Journal of Pediatrics, 39*(1), 30.

Güngör, D., Kruijshaar, M. E., Plug, I., D'Agostino, R. B., Hagemans, M. L., van Doorn, P. A., . . . van der Ploeg, A. T. (2013). Impact of enzyme replacement therapy on survival in adults with Pompe disease: Results from a prospective international observational study. *Orphanet Journal of Rare Diseases, 8*(1), 49.

Hagemans, M. L. C., Winkel, L. P. F., Hop, W. C. J., Reuser, A. J. J., Van Doorn, P. A., & Van der Ploeg, A. T. (2005). Disease severity in children and adults with Pompe disease related to age and disease duration. *Neurology, 64*(12), 2139–2141.

Hers, H. G. (1963). α-Glucosidase deficiency in generalized glycogen-storage disease (Pompe's disease). *Biochemical Journal, 86*(1), 11.

Hirschhorn, R., & Reuser, A. J. J. (2001). Glycogen storage disease type II; acid α-glucosidase (acid maltase) deficiency. In C. R. Scriver, A. L. Beaudet, W. Sly, & D. Valle, Eds. *The metabolic and molecular bases of inherited disease.* (Vol. III, pp. 3389–3420). New York, NY: McGraw-Hill.

Hobson-Webb, L. D., Jones, H. N., & Kishnani, P. S. (2013). Oropharyngeal dysphagia may occur in late-onset Pompe disease, implicating bulbar muscle involvement. *Neuromuscular Disorders, 23*(4), 319–323.

Jones, H. N., Crisp, K. D., Asrani, P., Sloane, R., & Kishnani, P. S. (2015). Quantitative assessment of lingual strength in late-onset Pompe disease. *Muscle & Nerve, 51*(5), 731–735.

Jones, H. N., Muller, C. W., Lin, M., Banugaria, S. G., Case, L. E., Li, J. S., . . . Kishnani, P. S. (2010). Oropharyngeal dysphagia in infants and children with infantile Pompe disease. *Dysphagia, 25*(4), 277–283.

Kishnani, P. S., & Beckemeyer, A. A. (2014). New therapeutic approaches for Pompe disease: Enzyme replacement therapy and beyond. *Pediatric Endocrinology Reviews: PER, 12,* 114–124.

Kishnani, P. S., Steiner, R. D., Bali, D., Berger, K., Byrne, B. J., Case, L. E., . . . Mackey, J. (2006). Pompe disease diagnosis and management guideline. *Genetics in Medicine, 8*(5), 267.

Lim, J. A., Li, L., & Raben, N. (2014). Pompe disease: From pathophysiology to therapy and back again. *Frontiers in Aging Neuroscience, 6,* 177.

Lin, C. Y., Hwang, B., Hsiao, K. J., & Jin, Y. R. (1987). Pompe's disease in Chinese and prenatal diagnosis by determination of α-glucosidase activity. *Journal of inherited metabolic disease, 10*(1), 11–17.

Lukacs, Z., Cobos, P. N., Wenninger, S., Willis, T. A., Guglieri, M., Roberts, M., . . . Schlotter-Weigel, B. (2016). Prevalence of Pompe disease in 3,076 patients with hyperCKemia and limb-girdle muscular weakness. *Neurology, 87*(3), 295–298.

Maggi, L., Salerno, F., Bragato, C., Saredi, S., Blasevich, F., Maccagnano, E., . . . Morandi, L. (2013). Familial adult-onset Pompe disease associated with unusual clinical and histological features. *Acta Myologica, 32*(2), 85.

Marsden, D. (2005). Infantile onset Pompe disease: A report of physician narratives from an epidemiologic study. *Genetics in Medicine, 7*(2), 147.

Martiniuk, F., Chen, A., Mack, A., Arvanitopoulos, E., Chen, Y., Rom, W. N., . . . & Plotz, P. (1998). Carrier frequency for glycogen storage disease type II in New York and estimates of affected individuals born with the disease. *American Journal of Medical Genetics, 79*(1), 69–72.

Meikle, P. J., Hopwood, J. J., Clague, A. E., & Carey, W. F. (1999). Prevalence of lysosomal storage disorders. *JAMA, 281*(3), 249–254.

National Organization for Rare Disorders. (2019). *Pompe disease.* Retrieved from https://rarediseases.org/rare-diseases/pompe-disease/

Pinto, R., Caseiro, C., Lemos, M., Lopes, L., Fontes, A., Ribeiro, H., . . . & Ribeiro, I. (2004). Prevalence of lysosomal storage diseases in Portugal. *European Journal of Human Genetics, 12*(2), 87.

Pompe, J. C. (1932). Over idiopathische hypertrophie van het hart. *Nederlands Tijdschrift voor Geneeskunde, 76,* 304–311.

12

Nemaline Myopathy

KEY WORDS: nemaline myopathy, scoliosis, congenital, nebulin, sarcomere

Definition

Nemaline myopathy (NM), also known as rod myopathy or nemaline rod myopathy, is a rare, **congenital**, hereditary neuro-muscular disorder. It is a disorder that mainly affects muscles, particularly the facial skeletal muscles. The muscular impairments are manifested in respiratory insufficiency, swallowing dysfunction, and motor speech disorders. Many individuals with NM also present with lower limb deformities, **scoliosis**, and joint deformities. The generalized myopathy often gets worse with the passage of time.

Myopathy means muscle disease. The muscle fibers from someone with NM contain threadlike rods called nemaline bodies (National Organization for Rare Diseases, 2016). It is believed that the presence of the rods is diagnostic of the disease, rather than causing a dysfunction on their own. Individuals with NM usually exhibit delayed motor development, or in severe cases, absent motor development. Weakness is present in all skeletal muscles such as the arms, legs, trunk, neck, throat, and face. The weakness is more severe in proximal muscles, as opposed to the more distal muscles.

Since muscle weakness of the face and neck is a main feature of NM, across most of the subtypes of NM, most individuals with this rare disease manifest some form of dysphagia.

There are six subtypes of NM. These are typical congenital myopathy (accounting for almost half of all cases), severe congenital, Amish, intermediate congenital, childhood onset, and adult onset (Table 12–1). Each subtype is distinguished by the age of onset.

Table 12–1. Characteristics of Nemaline Myopathy (NM) by Subtype

Subtype	Onset	Characteristics
Severe Congenital	Birth	Severe respiratory problems. Generalized hypotonia. Dysphagia: sucking and swallowing problems, gastroesophageal reflux. Low survival expectancy.
Amish Type	Birth	Hip contracture, motor delay, tremors, abnormality of rib cage, delayed motor development. Fatal in early childhood.
Intermediate Congenital	Birth	Ranges from mild to severe. Early joint contractures. Delayed motor development. Respiratory problems. Typically utilize wheelchair by early puberty.
Typical (Mild) Congenital	Birth–1 Year Old	Most common type of NM. Hypotonia. Severe muscle weakness. Severe feeding and swallowing problems. Better ambulation than other subtypes.

Table 12–1. *continued*

Subtype	Onset	Characteristics
Childhood Onset	8 Years Old–Adolescence	Muscle weakness manifested in adolescence. Slow, progressive weakness involving the ankles.
Adult Onset	20 Years Old–50 Years Old	Mildest of all types of NM. Generalized muscle weakness with pain. Proximal weakness. Respiratory difficulties. Sporadic occurrence with no family history of NM.

History

"Rod myopathy" is another associated term for nemaline myopathy. Australian physician Douglas Reye was the first person to identify this disease in 1958 through the biopsy of muscle tissue from one of his patients. Reye's report did not initially receive widespread attention. It wasn't until the turn of the 21st century when rod myopathy was confirmed in his patient (Schnell, Kan, & North, 2000). The term "nemaline myopathy" first gained public attention in a paper published in the early 1960s by North American researchers Cohen and Shy who discovered rodlike structures in the muscle fibers of patients diagnosed with muscle weakness (NORD, 2016).

Etiology

It is generally accepted that mutations of a variety of genes can cause NM. These genes provide instructions for producing the proteins that are critical to skeletal muscles. Within the cells of the skeletal muscles, the proteins are nestled in structures called

sarcomeres. Sarcomeres are important for muscle contraction. A microscopic examination of the skeletal muscle cells of individuals with NM reveals an abnormal appearance of these cells. It is in these abnormal muscle cells that the rodlike structures known as nemaline bodies appear.

Most NM cases with a known genetic source result from mutations in one of two genes, NEB or ACTA1. The NEB gene provides instructions for making a protein called **nebulin**. Nebulin is found in the sarcomeres and it is involved in the mechanical force needed for muscle contraction. The NEB gene mutations account for approximately 50% of all cases of NM, while ACTA1 gene mutations account for around 15% to 25% of all cases. When NM results from NEB mutations, the signs and symptoms of the disorder are often present at birth or in early childhood. On the other hand, when NM is caused by ACTA1 mutations, the severity of the condition and the age of onset tend to vary widely. Mutations in the other genes associated with NM account for a very small percentage of the cases (Lehtokari et al., 2006; Nowak et al., 2007).

NM is usually inherited in an autosomal *recessive* pattern. This means that both copies of the gene in each cell have mutations; that is, both parents of the person with an autosomal recessive pattern each carry one copy of the mutated gene, even though they have no symptoms of the disorder. A less inherited pattern is the autosomal *dominant* pattern. In this condition, one copy of the mutated gene in each is sufficient to cause the disorder. It is important to note that most cases of NM result from new mutations in the gene and occur in individuals with no history of the disorder in their family (NIH, 2019).

Epidemiology

NM is a rare disorder, the incidence of which is relatively unknown. But two studies—one in Finland and the other in the United States, both carried out in the American Ashkenazi Jewish population—estimated the incidence to be at 1 in 50,000 live births

(Anderson et al., 2004). Johnston et al. (2000) reported an incidence of 1 in 500 in the Amish community of the United States (NORD, 2016). In a review of 143 occurrences of NM in Australia and North America, Ryan et al. (2001) identified the frequency of occurrence of the different subtypes: severe congenital, 16%; intermediate congenital, 20%; typical congenital, 46%; childhood onset, 13%; and adult onset, 4%. This study also showed that the typical congenital subtype of NM was a more common occurrence compared to the other forms.

Clinical Presentation

The outstanding features of NM are muscle weakness, hypotonia, respiratory deficiency, limb deformities, and swallowing deficits. Muscle weakness tends to be more severe in the face, neck, and proximal limbs. The presence of prominent facial weakness as well as the generalized weakness and respiratory involvement are hallmark features of NM. The severity of weakness and disability varies widely, from neonates with profound generalized weakness to patients with subtle weakness that first manifests during childhood with delayed motor milestones, or even later in life with symptoms of proximal weakness (North et al., 2014). The most common mechanisms that appear to contribute to the feeding and swallowing problems experienced by individuals with NM are low muscle tone/muscle weakness and respiratory deficiencies.

Low Muscle Tone

The low muscle tone in the facial muscles seen in infants with NM often results in an open mouth posture. Under normal circumstances, stability of the jaw allows the tongue to dissociate movement patterns within the mouth; in the case of the open lax jaw, there is an immature anterior/posterior pattern of movement

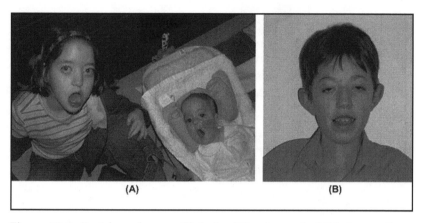

Figure 12–1. Facial weakness with lack of lip closure in NM. *Source*: From "Approach to the Diagnosis of Congenital Myopathies. Neuromuscular Disorders," by K. N. North, C. H. Wang, N. Clarke, H. Jungbluth, M. Vainzof, J. J. Dowling, . . . International Standard of Care Committee for Congenital Myopathies, 2014, *NMD, 24*(2), 97–116. doi:10.1016/j.nmd.2013.11.003

in which the tongue and the jaw move simultaneously (Manno, Fox, Eicher, & Kerwin, 2005). Furthermore, these wide excursions of the jaw compromise the ability to manipulate food inside the mouth, thus increasing the likelihood of either material falling out of the mouth or failure to chew smaller pieces of food. The lips and the cheeks in the unimpaired child work together, providing enough tension inside the mouth to contain the food. If the lip and cheek muscles are shortened due to compensatory motor movements, they will not be able to attain the full muscle length needed for lip closure (Figure 12–1). Consequently, low muscle tone of the oral structures can leave the lips in an open posture, eventually causing food to be lost anteriorly (Alper & Manno, 1996; Ernsperger & Stegen-Hanson, 2004).

Respiratory Insufficiency

As previously discussed, respiratory deficiency is a phenotype of NM. Sensory inputs from the respiratory and gastrointestinal tracts appear to have a direct influence on the oral motor patterns through the swallowing center in the brain stem (Miller, 1986). Since the upper respiratory tracts use the same structures as the upper digestive tracts (e.g., back of the mouth and pharynx), breathing is neurologically programmed to supersede feeding (Daniels, Devlieger, Minami, Eggermount, & Casaer, 1990). Therefore, any respiratory problems that make breathing more difficult will have a negative impact on feeding and swallowing.

Dysphagia and feeding problems appear in almost all subtypes of NM with varying degrees of severity. About 25% of individuals with the congenital NM will require gavage feeding or gastrostomy during the first few years of life (North & Ryan, 2015).

The clinical classification of NM into six subtypes reveals considerable overlap in the manifested signs and symptoms. This classification of subtypes is based on age of onset and severity of both motor and respiratory involvement.

Clinical Presentation—Severe Congenital NM (SCNM)

This form of NM is present at birth and accounts for at least 16% of cases. The affected infant presents with significant hypotonia and muscle weakness, with severely reduced to very little spontaneous movement. Infants with this subtype of NM usually present with remarkable sucking and swallowing difficulties, gastroesophageal reflux, and respiratory insufficiency (Figure 12–2). Typically, an infant with a congenital myopathy will not only be "floppy," but also have difficulty breathing and feeding, and will generally lag behind in development. SCNM is the subtype of NM with the most seriously involved sucking and swallowing problems leading to aspiration pneumonia that arises in utero.

During the pregnancy, the mother may report decreased fetal movements. In addition, the mother may also experience polyhydramnios that may further complicate the pregnancy. Polyhydramnios occurs when there is excess buildup of amniotic fluid during pregnancy. Amniotic fluid is the liquid that surrounds the baby in utero. The fluid is absorbed when the baby swallows it as well as through the motions of breathing. In the case of the

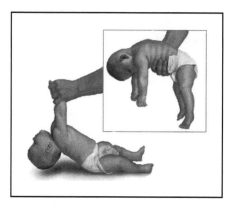

Figure 12–2. Floppy baby. *Source*: From "Neurological Phenotypes for Down Syndrome Across the Life Span," by I. T. Lott, 2012, *Progress in Brain Research, 197*, 101–121. doi.org/10.1016/B978-0-444-54299-1.00006-6

baby with SCNM, since there are reduced swallowing skills, the fluid often builds up. The reduced fetal movements as well as the polyhydramnios condition result in infant death in utero (Ryan et al., 2001). Early mortality secondary to respiratory insufficiency of aspiration pneumonia is common in this subtype of NM. However, even with the severe generalized hypotonia and poor respiratory ability, some infants still survive long term.

Clinical Presentation—Typical Congenital NM (TCNM)

TCNM is the most common form and accounts for approximately half of all cases. This form appears either at birth, shortly after, or during the first year of life. Most affected infants exhibit severe hypotonia that leads to floppiness as well as severe feeding problems. It must be noted that the muscle weakness in this type of NM is often less dramatic than in the severe congenital or the intermediate forms. It is not unusual for infants with TCNM to exhibit significant muscle weakness at birth that improves with age.

Infants with TCNM tend to experience weakness of respiratory muscles that inevitably leads to breathing problems. A common breathing problem is nocturnal hypoventilation. Nocturnal hypoventilation is a condition in which there is poor breathing during sleep that results in increased levels of carbon dioxide in the blood: a condition known as hypercarbia. Feeding and swallowing problems as well as dysarthric speech and abnormal gait are also present. These conditions are due to the pervasive muscle weakness present with NM.

Clinical Presentation—Amish NM (ANM)

Amish NM is a clinically distinct autosomal recessive form with neonatal onset and early childhood mortality (North et al., 2015). This subtype only appears in the Old Order Amish families (Johnston et al., 2000) as well as one reported case in a Dutch family (van der Pol et al., 2014). In the Old Order Amish families, their genetic origins and their strict endogamy predispose them to manifest rare disorders that are inherited in an autosomal recessive pattern (Johnston et al., 2000). In ANM disorder, infants in the first few months of life manifest tremors with hypotonia as well as shoulder and hip contractures. The progressive worsening of the contractures and respiratory distress contribute toward infant mortality within the second year of life. Typically, infants at birth present with hypotonia associated with contractures and tremors that tend to subside 2 to 3 months after birth. Not surprisingly, feeding and swallowing difficulties dominate ANM, but it is the progressive weakness and worsening respiratory insufficiency that ultimately lead to death in the second year of life.

Clinical Presentation—Intermediate Congenital NM (ICNM)

Intermediate congenital NM is less severe than the severe congenital form. Early development of joint contractures is the hallmark of this form of NM. Most individuals with ICNM exhibit generalized muscle weakness and severe muscular hypotonia (80%–99%). Still another 30% to 78% exhibit respiratory problems due to thoracic abnormality, difficulty walking, poor swallowing due to muscle weakness, and delay in the development of motor skills. A smaller percentage of cases (5%–29%) may exhibit facial diplegia, vaulted palate, and hypertelorism (wide set eyes). Most infants survive to the age of 11 when they manifest more severe respiratory and ambulatory difficulties (Genetics and Rare Diseases Information Center, 2011).

Clinical Presentation—Childhood-Onset NM (CONM)

This form of NM is usually more apparent around the first to second decade of life, and accounts for about 10% to 15% of all cases of NM. It is considered a milder form of NM. The onset tends to occur around 10 to 20 years of age, with the initial presentation of symmetric weakness of ankle dorsiflexion and foot drop (GARD, 2011). In CONM, muscle weakness tends to progress rather slowly. What differentiates it from the other subtypes is the fact that early motor development is normal. In the late first or early second decade, children manifest the onset of symmetric weakness of ankle dorsiflexion with foot drop. All the while, facial, respiratory, and cardiac muscles are generally normal. These patients are inhibited in movement activity such as running or jumping simply because of muscle weakness or slowness. Dysphagia is not a hallmark disorder in this subtype although some individuals may manifest the disorder depending on the severity of the subtype.

Clinical Presentation—Adult-Onset/Late-Onset NM (AONM)

AONM, sometimes referred to as sporadic late-onset nemaline myopathy, is a rapidly progressive type of NM. It occurs sporadically between 20 and 50 years of age (GARD, 2011). This subtype of NM varies in clinical presentation as well as in its progression. Most people with this phenotype exhibit generalized weakness without any prior manifestation of symptoms or hereditary source. Individuals with AONM present with cardiomyopathy, also referred to as "dropped head" syndrome. This syndrome creates weakness of neck extension with or without neck flexor weakness (Lomen-Hoerth, Simmons, Dearmond, & Layzer, 1999). Not surprisingly, many individuals with late onset NM exhibit dysphagia and dysarthria as the predominant clinical phenotype (Schnitzler et al., 2017).

Management of Dysphagia

Presently, no specific treatment exists for NM. However, treatment is supportive and geared toward the specific manifested symptoms that are apparent in each individual. Supportive mechanical ventilation; naso-gastric feeding; mobility aids; and physical, occupational, and speech therapy are major disciplines involved in the treatment protocols (Nowak, Davis, Wallgren-Pettersson, Lamont, & Laing, 2015).

Since the hallmark feature of NM is muscle weakness, it is conceivable that all forms of NM can have varying repercussions for swallowing. The obviously more severe subtypes such as the severe/neonatal congenital and the typical congenital tend to exhibit more severe feeding and swallowing disorders. Feeding disorders are problems with activities such as sucking, eating with a spoon, chewing, or drinking from a cup. Swallowing disorders, known as dysphagia, are related to abnormalities in any of the four phases of the normal swallowing mechanism, such as the oral preparatory, oral transport, pharyngeal, and esophageal phases (Arvedson, Clark, Lazarus, Schooling, & Frymark, 2010).

Assessment

In infants and children who present with either feeding or swallowing problems, an in-depth swallowing assessment, usually performed by the speech-language pathologist (SLP), is needed so that the appropriate management and recommendations for adequate and safe feeding can be made. The assessment should include taking an inventory of feeding and swallowing problems, observing eating and drinking of different consistencies, and, perhaps most importantly, assessing the neuromotor development and oral motor skills (van den Engel-Hoek, de Groot, de Swart, & Erasmus, 2015).

Swallowing in children and adults is different in that the anatomy of the oral structures is different (Figure 12–3). Consequently, the consistency of the food and the manner of delivery will also be different.

The common factor in most cases of NM previously discussed is muscle weakness. This will significantly impact motor skills as well as oral motor activities. For example, in assessing the feeding or swallowing skills of the infant, variables such as (1) the onset of swallowing problems, (2) the phases of the swallowing problem, and (3) the throat muscle involvement should be carefully examined.

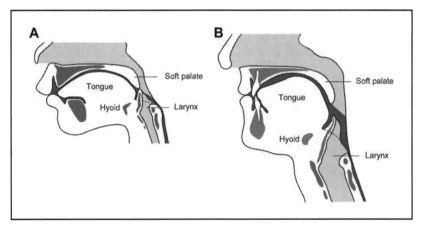

Figure 12–3. Anatomy of oral structures in the infant (A) compared to the adult (B). *Source*: Adapted from "Anatomy and Physiology of Feeding and Swallowing: Normal and Abnormal," by K. Matsuo and J. B. Palmer, 2008, *Physical Medicine and Rehabilitation Clinics of North America, 19*(4), 691–707.

Onset of Swallowing Problems

As previously discussed, fetal dysphagia tends to occur in the most serious subtypes of NM. This type of dysphagia occurs in relation to polyhydramnios. Feeding difficulties may occur at birth and are usually related to a weak or underdeveloped sucking pattern. Sometimes the infant with NM may exhibit coughing during feeding. This may be due to some residue in the pharynx post swallow. It is extremely important for the SLP to perform a thorough assessment in order to make the correct feeding decision. Infants with a weak swallow may have greater difficulty managing thicker liquids as this viscosity requires stronger suction and could therefore worsen the problem with pharyngeal residue. If the sucking and swallowing are not only weak but also utterly impossible, it may be necessary for a feeding tube to be placed so that the infant can obtain adequate nutrition.

In some cases of NM, chewing difficulties can emerge as a later symptom of dysphagia. Some of the signs of this complication are extended mealtimes, or even episodes of choking and poor nutritional intake. In some cases where the myopathy gets worse, even though the child may be able to chew, the problem is exacerbated due to weakness of the facial muscles such as the masseter and the temporal muscles; in addition, weakened tongue movement can create reduced oral propulsion—all of which can lead to material collecting throughout the pharynx.

The Phases of the Swallowing Problem

Weakened oral muscles have a significant impact on the oral preparatory phase of the swallow. This weakness can affect both sucking and mastication. Even if the infant's nutritional problem is solved by the provision of tube feedings, the downside to this is that it prevents the infant from developing the muscles involved in oral feeding. In NM children, the oral phase of the swallow is often met with impairments such as limited mouth opening, tented upper lip, and high arched palate. Many NM children exhibit drooling due to open mouth posture, reduced tongue movement, as well as reduced subconscious swallowing frequency. Typically, upon examination of the oral musculature as well as the oral phase of the swallow, the speech-language pathologist will observe piecemeal deglutition manifested in the form of multiple swallows and poor bolus formation (material scattered throughout the oral cavity), notably post swallow.

At the pharyngeal phase, typically observed via videofluoroscopy (VFSS), the problems can range from nasal regurgitation to residue in the pharyngeal pockets (valleculae, pyriforms) as well as on the pharyngeal wall post swallow that eventually lead to laryngeal penetration and aspiration. A major difficulty that most NM patients face is reduced pharyngeal pressure during swallow as well as reduced relaxation of the upper esophageal sphincter (UES). This difficulty is most often due to weakness of the submental muscle group (Weir, McMahon, Taylor, & Chang, 2011).

Residue above the UES post swallow is a common observation in the NM patient. This residue may occur because of either a pharyngeal or an esophageal dysmotility. The esophageal motor problems are directly related to the hypotonicity and weakness of the UES, which often lead to reduced esophageal peristalsis and thus retention of material in the esophagus post swallow. The cyclic effect is regurgitation of the retained material from the esophagus into the pharynx, with the risk of aspiration (van den Engel-Hoek et al., 2015).

In managing the swallowing issues that children with NM face, the SLP must bear in mind that children with NM very often do not gain experience with feeding in the neonatal stage. This is because the feeding problem is usually so severe that alternative feeding (tube-feedings) have to be the primary mode of nutrition for survival. Consequently, as the infant thrives, oral feeding has to be introduced gradually. Very careful introduction of small amounts of liquid and solids must be monitored. Van den Engel-Hoek et al. (2015) suggest introduction of oral simultaneous with tube feeding (Seguy et al., 2002).

Treatment of swallowing problems in NM requires the SLP to be knowledgeable of the fact that there is still a wide variety of dysphagia symptoms even across the various subtypes of NM. For example, it is known that in the severe congenital form, NM infants present with the most severe inability to suck and swallow, leading to aspiration pneumonia. Those who survive have to be fed in many cases via gastrostomy. Treating oral feeding skills in these infants requires the approach to be one of facilitating the development of skills that were never present. On the other hand, there are those individuals with other subtypes of NM—for example, childhood and adult onset—whose symptoms emerge after they had already acquired swallowing skills. In the childhood onset, the symptoms of the disorder (muscle weakness) appear in the first to second decade of life and the progression is slow. Dysphagia in this type is usually milder and tends to be oropharyngeal, especially for solid textures. In the adult onset, the symptoms of NM emerge between 20 and 50 years of age and the symptoms of dysphagia appear more so in the oropharyngeal and upper esophageal regions. This knowledge of the time of onset and the nature of dysphagia symptoms is critical in planning treatment protocols.

The differences in the nature of the feeding and swallowing problems call for careful assessment by way of clinical and instrumental swallow studies to establish the nature of the problem. Since not all cases of NM will present in the exact same manner, treatment of feeding and swallowing must be tailored to each specific case. In the case of sucking and swallowing problems in the neonatal onset of NM, a nasogastric tube may be used to supplement the diet if nutritional needs are not being met adequately (van den Engel-Hoek et al., 2015). In some cases, infants with NM may benefit from mild to moderate low-impact exercises, massage, and stretching techniques (NORD, 2016).

Management of dysphagia in individuals with NM of any subtype will require collaboration of a multidisciplinary team: neurologist, speech-language pathologist, physical therapist, occupational therapist, respiratory therapist, and dietician. There is still a lot more that needs to be unpacked regarding this rather rare and intriguing disorder of nemaline myopathy. As more research is carried out regarding the nature of the disorder and its subtypes, more innovative approaches to treatment will emerge.

Summary

Nemaline myopathy is a rare, congenital, hereditary disorder that mainly affects the skeletal muscles, which are those muscles that are primarily involved in movement. The hallmark of NM is muscle weakness (myopathy) throughout the body, but it is typically most severe in the muscles of the face, neck, trunk, as well as the upper arms and legs. Individuals with NM usually present with feeding and swallowing problems, severe respiratory insufficiencies, foot deformities, scoliosis, and a multiplicity of contractures. Many patients with NM may still be able to walk, although some affected children will be developmentally delayed. As the NM progresses, some individuals will need wheelchair assistance. In severe presentations of NM, some patients may manifest severe, life-threatening respiratory difficulties.

There are six subtypes of NM: severe congenital (SCNM), Amish (ANM), intermediate congenital (ICNM), typical congenital (TCNM), childhood onset (CONM), and adult onset (AONM). These various types are distinguished by the age and severity of the symptoms, even though there may be an overlap of the symptoms in the different subtypes. Nevertheless, SCNM is regarded as the worst of these subtypes. Many individuals with SCNM do not typically survive past early childhood because of respiratory complications. ANM subtype has only been reported in Old Order Amish families of Pennsylvania and in at least one Dutch family. Patients with ANM also do not survive past early childhood. The TCNM type of NM is the most commonly reported type. Feeding and swallowing problems along with muscle weakness in early childhood are prominent in this subtype. The remarkable characteristic of this type is that most of the individuals do not suffer with respiratory problems and are able to walk without assistance. In the CONM subtype, the myopathy with all of the accompanying effects such as gait and swallowing deficits usually emerge during adolescence. The sixth subtype, AONM, usually manifests the myopathies of NM between the ages of 20 and 50 years of age.

There is no specific cure for the disease; however, treatment is supportive and is aimed at the specific symptoms manifested in each individual. In terms of feeding and swallowing, the goal of treatment is to minimize pulmonary problems secondary to aspiration and to maximize adequate nutrition. Treatment is best when rendered from a multidisciplinary approach.

References

Alper, B. S., & Manno, C. J. (1996). Dysphagia in infants and children with oral-motor deficits: Assessment and management. *Seminars in Speech and Language, 17*(4), 283–310.

Anderson, S. L., Ekstein, J., Donnelly, M. C., Keefe, E. M., Toto, N. R., LeVoci, L. A., & Rubin, B. Y. (2004). Nemaline myopathy in the Ashkenazi Jewish population is caused by a deletion in the nebulin gene. *Human Genetics, 115*(3), 185–190.

Arvedson, J., Clark, H., Lazarus, C., Schooling, T., & Frymark, T. (2010). Evidence-based systematic review: Effects of oral motor interventions on feeding and swallowing in preterm infants. *American Journal of Speech-Language Pathology, 19*(4), 321–340.

Daniels, H., Devlieger, H., Minami, T., Eggermont, E., & Casaer, P. (1990). Infant feeding and cardiorespiratory maturation. *Neuropediatrics, 21*(1), 9–10.

Ernsperger, L., & Stegen-Hanson, T. (2004). *Just take a bite: Easy, effective answers to food aversions and eating challenges!* Arlington, TX. Future Horizons.

Genetic and Rare Diseases Information Center [GARD]. (2011). *Intermediate congenital nemaline myopathy.* Retrieved from https://rarediseases.info.nih.gov/diseases/12823/intermediate-congenital-nemaline-myopathy

Johnston, J. J., Kelley, R. I., Crawford, T. O., Morton, D. H., Agarwala, R., Koch, T., . . . Biesecker, L. G. (2000). A novel nemaline myopathy in the

Amish caused by a mutation in troponin T1. *American Journal of Human Genetics, 67*(4), 814–821.

Lehtokari, V. L., Pelin, K., Sandbacka, M., Ranta, S., Donner, K., Muntoni, F., . . . Iannaccone, S. (2006). Identification of 45 novel mutations in the nebulin gene associated with autosomal recessive nemaline myopathy. *Human Mutation, 27*(9), 946–956.

Lomen-Hoerth, C., Simmons, M. L., Dearmond, S. J., & Layzer, R. B. (1999). Adult-onset nemaline myopathy: Another cause of dropped head. *Muscle & Nerve: Official Journal of the American Association of Electrodiagnostic Medicine, 22*(8), 1146–1150.

Lott, I. T. (2012). Neurological phenotypes for Down syndrome across the life span. *Progress in Brain Research, 197*, 101–121. doi.org/10.1016 /B978-0-444-54299-1.00006-6

Manno, C. J., Fox, C., Eicher, P. S., & Kerwin, M. E. (2005). Early oral-motor interventions for pediatric feeding problems: What, when and how. *Journal of Early and Intensive Behavior Intervention, 2*(3), 145.

Matsuo, K., & Palmer, J. B. (2008). Anatomy and physiology of feeding and swallowing: Normal and abnormal. *Physical Medicine and Rehabilitation Clinics of North America, 19*(4), 691–707.

Miller, A. J. (1986). Neurophysiological basis of swallowing. *Dysphagia, 1*(2), 91.

National Organization for Rare Diseases [NORD]. (2016). *Nemaline myopathy*. Retrieved from https://rarediseases.org/rare-diseases/nemaline -myopathy/

NIH. (2019). *U.S. National Library of Medicine*. Retrieved January 29, 2019, from https://ghr.nlm.nih.gov.

North, K. N., & Ryan, M. M. (2015). Nemaline myopathy. In *Gene Reviews®[Internet]*. Seattle, WA: University of Washington.

North, K. N., Wang, C. H., Clarke, N., Jungbluth, H., Vainzof, M., Dowling, J. J., . . . Laing, N. G. (2014). Approach to the diagnosis of congenital myopathies. *Neuromuscular Disorders, 24*(2), 97–116.

Nowak, K. J., Davis, M. R., Wallgren-Pettersson, C., Lamont, P. J., & Laing, N. G. (2015). Clinical utility gene card for: Nemaline myopathy– Update 2015. *European Journal of Human Genetics, 23*(11), 1588.

Nowak, K. J., Sewry, C. A., Navarro, C., Squier, W., Reina, C., Ricoy, J. R., . . . Mountford, R. C. (2007). Nemaline myopathy caused by absence of α-skeletal muscle actin. *Annals of Neurology: Official Journal of the American Neurological Association and the Child Neurology Society, 61*(2), 175–184.

Ryan, M. M., Schnell, C., Strickland, C. D., Shield, L. K., Morgan, G., Iannaccone, S. T., . . . North, K. N. (2001). Nemaline myopathy: A clinical study of 143 cases. *Annals of Neurology: Official Journal of the American Neurological Association and the Child Neurology Society, 50*(3), 312–320.

Schnell, C., Kan, A., & North, K. N. (2000). An artefact gone awry. In "Identification of the First Case of Nemaline Myopathy" by R. D. K. Reye. *Neuromuscular Disorders, 10*(4–5), 307–312.

Schnitzler, L. J., Schreckenbach, T., Nadaj-Pakleza, A., Stenzel, W., Rushing, E. J., Van Damme, P., . . . Meisel, A. (2017). Sporadic late-onset nemaline myopathy: Clinico-pathological characteristics and review of 76 cases. *Orphanet Journal of Rare Diseases, 12*(1), 86.

Seguy, D., Michaud, L., Guimber, D., Cuisset, J. M., Devos, P., Turck, D., & Gottrand, F. (2002). Efficacy and tolerance of gastrostomy feeding in pediatric forms of neuromuscular diseases. *Journal of Parenteral and Enteral Nutrition, 26*(5), 298–304.

van den Engel-Hoek, L., de Groot, I. J., de Swart, B. J., & Erasmus, C. E. (2015). Feeding and swallowing disorders in pediatric neuromuscular diseases: An overview. *Journal of Neuromuscular Diseases, 2*(4), 357–369.

van der Pol, W. L., Leijenaar, J. F., Spliet, W. G., Lavrijsen, S. W., Jansen, N. J., Braun, K. P., . . . van Haelst, M. M. (2014). Nemaline myopathy caused by TNNT1 mutations in a Dutch pedigree. *Molecular Genetics & Genomic Medicine, 2*(2), 134–137.

Weir, K. A., McMahon, S., Taylor, S., & Chang, A. B. (2011). Oropharyngeal aspiration and silent aspiration in children. *Chest, 140*(3), 589–597.

13

Immunoglobulin
G4-Related Disease

KEY WORDS: immunoglobulin, extra-pyramidal dyskinesia, athetosis, thyroiditis, odynophagia, arytenoids, corticosteroids

Definition

Immunoglobulin G4-related disease (IgG4-RD) is a protean condition that mimics many malignant, infectious, and inflammatory disorders. IgG4-RD is a multiorgan, immune-mediated condition; it links many disorders previously regarded as isolated, single-organ diseases without any known underlying systemic condition (Kamisawa, Zen, Pillai & Stone, 2015). IgG4-RD is a relatively rare immune-mediated fibroinflammatory disorder that involves numerous organ sites; most organs, with the exception of the brain parenchyma, are affected by IgG4-RD (Caruthers, Khosroshahi, Augustin, Deshpande, & Stone, 2015).

Immunoglobulins, also known as antibodies, are glycoprotein molecules produced by the white blood cells. (Khosroshahi et al., 2015). These antibodies serve as a critical part of the immune system's response to fight against bacteria or viruses. In IgG4-RD, cells in the blood produce harmful substances that attack the body's own tissues, causing inflammation, swelling, and scarring in multiple organs (Casian & D'Cruz, 2016). Several presentations of the disease may be manifested in the salivary glands, lacrimal glands, thyroid gland, lymph nodes, and soft tissue of the neck, ear, and sinonasal tract. The underlying pathophysiological mechanism of IgG4-RD is still unclear, and if untreated, the disease can lead to irreversible organ damage (Karim et al., 2016).

Three classical features of IgG4-RD include masses that may eventually form tumors, collection of plasma cells, and elevated serum IgG4 levels that may affect virtually every organ and tissue of the body (Al-Mujaini, Al-Khabori, Shenoy, & Wali, 2018). The masses can often impinge on nerves or blood vessels, causing vascular or neurological problems. Single or multiple organs can be involved in IgG4-RD. Localized masses and/or nodules can occur in the kidneys and lungs, or there may be diffuse enlargement of an organ such as the pancreas.

IgG4-RD is included in this book because of its rarity as well as the emerging links to dysphagia that are now being reported. Of significance to speech-language pathologists is the fact that IgG4-RD affects organs such as the salivary glands, esophagus, as well as the thyroid. Involvement of these structures can negatively affect the process of swallowing, as will be discussed further in this chapter.

History

Long before IgG4-RD was fully described, there were reports about inflammatory disorders of the liver, bile ducts, and gall bladder. Although patients with these conditions have been described more than 100 years ago, the systemic nature of IgG4-RD has only just been recognized in the 21st century. However, the earliest description of IgG4-RD can be traced back to 1892, when Johann Mikulicz (Pieringer et al., 2014) described a patient with an inflammatory disease of the salivary glands (Mikulicz syndrome). Later, in 1896, Kuttner described a patient with a tumorlike lesion of the submandibular glands (Pieringer et al., 2014). Later on, cases were described of an autoimmune, steroid-responsive form of pancreatitis (Yoshida et al., 1995), now known as type 1 autoimmune pancreatic (AIP), another synonym for IgG4-RD. Hamano et al. (2001) subsequently described a form of pancreatitis that was not related to that found in patients with a history of alcohol abuse. These researchers described the disorder in which not only pancreatitis was present but also fibrous tissue in other visceral organs. This was the first recognition of IgG4-RD as a multiorgan disorder. It was as recently as 2012 that the unified nomenclature IgG4-RD was used to encompass these various conditions. Around this same period, a Japanese research group established diagnostic criteria for IgG4-RD, thus creating international consensus for the disorder (Okazaki & Umehara, 2012).

Etiology

The etiology of IgG4-RD is largely unknown, even though the evidence clearly supports an autoimmune basis. Ascertaining the specific cause of the disorder is problematic because of the multiple organ involvement. Recent studies have suggested a possible link between IgG4-RD and environmental factors such as solvents, industrial and metal dusts, as well as certain pigments used in oils (de Buy Wenniger, Culver, & Beuers, 2014). These researchers found that the majority of their patients surveyed who had a diagnosis of IgG4-RD were blue-collar workers who work in areas such as building construction and plumbing. However, the environmental link to IgG4-RD requires further investigation.

Epidemiology

A few studies have reported on the epidemiology of IgG4-RD, but the majority of these reports are derived from Asian research. In

2009, a Japanese study estimated 800 individuals with IgG4-RD, thus accounting for a prevalence of 60 in 1,000,000 with IgG4-RD (Pieringer et al., 2014). More males have been reported with IgG4-RD compared to females. The prevalence rates in Western countries have not yet been fully established. However (Inoue et al., 2015), concluded that IgG4-RD is an adult disease with about 90% of patients over 50 years of age, although rare pediatric cases have been reported. Most studies report an overall predilection for the male sex, especially for IgG4-related pancreatitis, with a male to female ratio of 3:7. However, it is interesting that male and female patients differ in the affected organ manifestations. For example, IgG4-RD with infection of the salivary glands (sialadenitis) and infection of the tear duct (dacryoadenitis) tends to be more prevalent in females. Most patients with infected salivary glands have trouble in the oral preparatory stage of the swallow. Although IgG4-RD can involve various organs, 60% of patients have pancreatitis, suggesting that pancreatitis is a prototypic manifestation of IgG4-RD.

The few reports that address epidemiology in IgG4-RD suggest a high occurrence in Asian patients, but this is by no means definitive. Traditionally, IgG4-related pancreatitis is regarded as the most frequent manifestation of IgG4-RD. European, American, and Asian patients differ not only in the overall prevalence of IgG4-RD, but also in the frequency of certain organ manifestations.

Clinical Presentation

IgG4-RD is comprised of a collection of disorders that share particular pathologic, serologic, and clinical features (Kamisawa et al., 2015; Stone, Zen, & Deshpande, 2012). Many conditions can mimic IgG4-RD (Table 13–1), hence the importance of a full clinical history, physical examination, selected laboratory investigations, and appropriate radiological studies.

The presentation of IgG4-RD is challenging because the number of diseases associated with the disorder continues to

Table 13–1. Some Common Conditions That Mimic IgG4-RD

Condition	Description
Granulomatosis with Polyangiitis	Inflammation of the blood vessels
Adenocarcinoma	Type of cancer that commonly starts in mucous gland in organs such as the lungs, colon, and breast
Castleman's Disease	Proliferation of cells in the lymph nodes
Inflammatory Myofibroblastic Tumor	Benign tumor found in young people, occurs anywhere in the body but mostly in the lungs, eye-socket, lining of internal organs
Inflammatory Bowel Disease	Group of intestinal disorders causing inflammation of the digestive tract
Primary Sclerosing Cholangitis	Progressive liver and gallbladder disease characterized by scarring and inflammation of the bile ducts, common cause of cirrhosis
Rhinosinusitis	Inflammation of nasal passages and sinuses
Rosai-Dorfman Disease	Accumulation of white cells in the lymph nodes most commonly in the neck region.
Sarcoidosis	Inflammatory cells/granulomas that grow anywhere in the body but most often in the lungs or lymph nodes
Sjogren's Syndrome	Immune system disorder, common symptoms dry eyes and dry mouth

grow (Carruthers, Stone, Deshpande, & Khosroshahi, 2012). Furthermore, the clinical presentation of IgG4-RD depends largely on the organs that are involved. Although symptoms may sometimes be mild, it can also cause severe organ damage and even death if not treated.

Classic clinical manifestations of IgG4-RD are autoimmune pancreatitis (AIP) type 1, which involves the major salivary glands.

Lesions of the salivary glands can appear as enlargements or inflammation that often form tumors. The disease frequently affects the eyes (most often in women), retroperitoneum (inside of the belly around the aorta, the largest blood vessel), gallbladder, kidneys, cranial nerves, and any organ of the body—thus creating a host of disorders that may otherwise appear to be unrelated. One major disorder that results from IgG4-RD is dysphagia. This results primarily when organs such as the *salivary glands, thyroid, esophagus,* as well as some *cranial nerves* become affected. These organs will be discussed in terms of their implication in dysphagia in the following sections.

Functions of Saliva

Saliva is derived mainly from three paired major salivary glands. These are the parotid, submandibular, and sublingual glands as well as minor salivary glands located in the oral mucosa.

Saliva has multiple functions, some of these are cleansing of the oral cavity, solubilization of food material to aid in bolus formation, mastication, and swallowing. For example, food in the mouth initiates mechanical and chemical stimuli by way of neural reflexes that result in a flow of saliva within the oral cavity (Table 13–2); these actions occur during the oral preparatory and oral phases of the swallow (Nauntofte & Jensen, 1999). In addition, saliva serves to lubricate the oral mucosa and to facilitate the smooth movements of the speech articulators (Pedersen, Bardow, Jensen, & Nauntofte, 2002). Furthermore, some of the components of saliva are not only essential to the coating of the oral mucosa, but to the digestive process.

Saliva plays a major role in maintaining the lubrication, clearance, and buffering of the oral, oropharyngeal, and esophageal mucosa. The saliva at this level is produced mainly by the submandibular, sublingual, and minor salivary glands (Pedersen et al., 2002). Consequently, any disorders of the salivary glands present in IgG4-RD will affect the salivary function and thus interfere with the integrity of the entire process of swallowing.

Table 13–2. Common Clinical Findings in Salivary Dysfunction

Clinical Presentation	Manifested Symptoms
Atrophic dry oral mucosa	Oral mucosa soreness and dryness
Fissured appearance of tongue	Tongue adherence to palate
Oral infections	Burning oral sensation
Increased dental caries	Food sticking to dental surfaces
Pharyngitis, laryngitis	Dysphonia
Atrophy masticatory muscles	Difficulty in mastication
Esophagitis	Acid reflux
Dry mucosa	Bad breath

Some individuals with salivary gland dysfunction, such as swollen parotid and or submandibular glands, often present with symptoms such as dry oral mucosa, burning oral sensation, difficulty swallowing, or disturbed mastication.

Thyroid

Movement of the laryngeal structures facilitates normal swallowing. In human beings, the larynx is comprised of nine cartilages: epiglottis, thyroid, cricoid, paired **arytenoids**, corniculates, and cuneiforms. These are all held together by muscles, membranes, and ligaments. During a normal swallow, particularly at the oral and pharyngeal phases, the larynx is lifted upward and forward. Failure of the larynx to elevate can lead to aspiration of material into the airway. Many circumstances can conspire to reduce laryngeal elevation. The most common cause is neurological, although mechanical conditions—that is, any condition that obstructs the elevation of the larynx—may also contribute.

Thyroiditis is inflammation of the thyroid gland. This gland is located in the region of the thyroid cartilage. Thyroiditis results from various conditions, among these are autoimmune, inflammatory, and drug-induced disorders. One type of thyroiditis that has been reported in some patients with IgG4-RD is Hashimoto's thyroiditis (HT), also referred to a IgG4-RD HT. HT is a type of thyroid disorder that is characterized by inflammation of the thyroid gland, IgG4-RD plasma cells, and significant fibrosis (Luiz et al., 2014). These researchers reported the case of a 56-year-old male with inflammation of his thyroid gland. The progressive swelling in his neck caused significant dysphagia. Further testing revealed positive IgG4-RD with Hashimoto's thyroiditis. It is good to recognize that any swelling in the neck area will not only interfere with the elevation of the larynx during the swallow, but can also compress the esophagus, thus restricting the esophageal phase of the swallow.

Esophagus

For descriptive purposes, the swallowing process is usually divided into four phases: the preparatory phase, the oral phase, the pharyngeal phase, and the esophageal phase. The preparatory phase and the oral phase are considered to be under voluntary control, whereas the pharyngeal and esophageal phases are under involuntary control.

The passage of the pharyngeal contraction to the upper esophageal sphincter signals transition from the pharyngeal phase to the esophageal phase of the swallow. Normally, the passage of the bolus through the esophagus, which is about 20 cm in length and takes about 6 to 10 s depending on the food texture and viscosity (Dodds, 1989). Disorders of the esophagus often lead to dysphagia regardless of the etiology of the disorder. Any disorder that alters the tissue, size, or contraction of the esophagus will lead to dysphagic symptoms.

Patients with IgG4-RD typically present with tumefactive lesions in several organs. Recent studies have revealed the involvement of the esophagus in a number of patients (Obiorah et al., 2017). Individuals with esophagitis usually present with dysphagia for solid foods, manifested in occasional pain and even vomiting. Obiorah et al. described the symptoms of dysphagia in patients with esophagitis secondary to a diagnosis of IgG4-RD. These patients exhibited esophageal strictures, erosive esophagitis, and esophageal nodules.

Early cases of esophageal dysphagia related to IgG4-RD were reported by Oh et al. (2015). These researchers noted progressive dysphagia in a 33-year-old male due to a mass in the cervical esophagus and multifocal calcified lymph nodes in the lower neck. Fiberoptic endoscopic evaluation of the swallow (FEES) revealed residue in the pyriform bilaterally but less so in the valleculae, suggesting some involvement at the level of the cricopharyngeal region.

Generally, the clinical symptoms of esophageal disorders include dysphagia, **odynophagia**, and weight loss, symptoms that are evident in most patients with esophagitis secondary to IgG4-RD.

Esophagitis is now being recognized as a phenotype of IgG4-RD. Lopes, Hochwald, Lancia, Dixon, and Ben-David (2010) presented a case of a 23-year-old male whose first clinical signs were dysphagia, weight loss, and recurrent esophageal strictures. Further endoscopic evaluation revealed the presence of a tumor in the distal esophagus. According to these researchers, the esophagitis was the first report as part of the IgG4-RD spectrum of diseases.

Cranial Nerves

Several cranial nerves individually and collectively are involved in different aspects of the swallowing process (Table 13–3). The swallow-related motor output to the musculature is transmitted to the muscles of the pharynx and esophagus. Muscles for mastication receive innervation from the mandibular branch of the trigeminal nerve (CV), while the hypoglossal nerve (XII) controls tongue movement. On the other hand, the vagus nerve (X) innervates the larynx, pharynx, palate, and esophagus. Damage to any of these nerves can negatively affect a person's ability to swallow safely (see Table 13–3).

Table 13–3. Cranial Nerves Involved in Swallowing

Cranial Nerve	Motor	Sensory	Swallowing Impairment
VII Facial	Muscles of the face	Taste sensation to anterior two-thirds of tongue	Reduced taste, spillage due to poor lip closure
V Trigeminal	Muscles of mastication	Touch sensation to soft palate—entire mouth, anterior two-thirds of tongue, nasopharynx	Oral prep, bolus spillage, decreased chewing residual in oral cavity
XII Hypoglossal	Intrinsic muscles of tongue		Apraxia of swallow, poor bolus formation, reduced tongue strength, oral residue
X Vagus	Palate, pharynx, larynx, & esophagus	Touch sensation to root of tongue, interior larynx	Reduced laryngeal elevation, nasal regurgitation, episodes of choking sensation
IX Glossopharyngeal	Pharynx	Taste sensation to posterior one-third of tongue	Reduced taste, decreased gag reflex

IgG4-RD is a recognized immune-mediated condition that affects a multiplicity of organs including the cranial nerves. Consequently, it is important to consider the role of the cranial nerves in the swallowing process. As discussed elsewhere, in IgG4-RD, the classic features include swellings that usually form tumors, collection of plasma cells, and elevated serum IgG4 levels. The swellings or masses can press on nerves or blood vessels, producing focal vascular and/or neurologic deficits (Al-Mujaini et al., 2018).

Even though, in the condition of IgG4-RD, nerve damage can be derived from tumors pressing on the specific nerve, this is not as frequently reported in the literature. This may be because IgG4-RD is still relatively new. However, Wallace et al. (2013) reported the case of a 52-year-old woman who presented with recurrent dysarthria, right facial weakness and numbness, dysphagia, and gait deficits. Neurological examination revealed deficits to cranial nerves VII, VIII, X, and XII. She was subsequently diagnosed with IgG4-RD.

Katsura, Morita, Horiuchi, Ohtomo, and Machida (2011) presented the case of IgG4-RD trigeminal nerve damage secondary to tumor. They suggested that trigeminal nerve tumor might be a component of IgG4-RD. Generally, the case for dysphagia in IgG4-RD so far can only be made based on the opportunistic involvement of the particular organ involved.

Management of Dysphagia

IgG4-RD is a relatively new disease entity and its natural history and clinical histopathology is still very unclear. Consequently, management of the disorder can be a major challenge since it depends on careful identification of the organs that may be involved. An additional challenge is the fact that clinical presentation of the disorder is not readily distinguishable from other disorders because it tends to mimic other diseases. Nevertheless, if diagnosed early, the potential for reversibility of clinical glandular function, for example, is known to be very good. This is particularly true in the case of manifested inflamed salivary glands (Shimizu et al., 2012). In this study, Shimizu et al. found that there was an improvement in salivary secretion following treatments with prednisolone. In this case, once the saliva improved, obviously, dysphagia secondary to dry mouth would also improve.

Patients with IgG4-RD tend to have a very positive response to **corticosteroids**. Based on reports in the literature, most cases of esophageal dysphagia secondary to IgG4-RD appear to improve with corticosteroid treatment. Oh et al. (2015) described a case of a patient with esophageal dysphagia due to IgG4-RD. FEES showed a large amount of residue at both pyriform recesses and relatively less residue at the valleculae, as well as hypercontraction in the upper esophageal region. This patient was treated with corticosteroid medication and prednisolone, and eventually all dysphagia symptoms were alleviated.

For the most part, management of dysphagia in IgG4-RD, as in most cases of rare diseases, is symptom specific. This means that there is no broad-brush approach to treatment. While the speech-language pathologist may provide appropriate management strategies to alleviate the dysphagia symptoms or to decrease the occurrence of aspiration, in many cases, when the underlying cause of the dysphagia is treated, more often than not, the swallowing problem is greatly relieved. The current consensus in treating IgG4-RD is that once an accurate diagnosis is made of the disease and intervention occurs early, the disease is highly amenable to medical intervention, particularly corticosteroids.

Summary

IgG4-RD is a rare, chronic inflammatory condition that is characterized by elevated serum levels of IgG4, infiltration of IgG4-positive plasmacytes, and storiform fibrosis in a variety of body organs. The etiology of the disease is largely unknown, but it is widely believed that it is autoimmune mediated. There is also a possible link between IgG4-RD and environmental factors such as solvents, industrial and metal dusts, as well as certain pigments used in oils (de Buy Wenniger et al., 2013).

IgG4-RD was recently recognized in the 21st century—even though its earliest description can be traced back to 1892, when Johann Mikulicz (Pieringer et al., 2014) described a patient with an inflammatory disease of the salivary glands, subsequently known as Mikulicz syndrome. IgG4-RD has a progressive clinical course. Tumorlike masses that tend to be fibrotic are the predominant clinical characteristics of the disease. Even though any organ of the body can be affected, the main organs implicated that might be of significance for dysphagia are the salivary glands, thyroid gland, esophagus, and compression any cranial nerve involved in the swallowing process. Currently, the most effective treatment for IgG4-RD consists of steroids and immunosuppressants. Interestingly, some studies have demonstrated that effective response to the steroids therapy tends to result in improvement of the dysphagia symptoms.

References

Al-Mujaini, A., Al-Khabori, M., Shenoy, K., & Wali, U. (2018). Immunoglobulin G4-related disease: An update. *Oman Medical Journal, 33*(2), 97.

de Buy Wenniger, L. J. M., Culver, E. L., & Beuers, U. (2013). Exposure to occupational antigens might predispose to IgG4-related disease. *Hepatology, 57*(6), 2390–2398.

Carruthers, M. N., Khosroshahi, A., Augustin, T., Deshpande, V., & Stone, J. H. (2015). The diagnostic utility of serum IgG4 concentrations in IgG4-related disease. *Annals of the Rheumatic Diseases, 74*(1), 14–18.

Carruthers, M. N., Stone, J. H., Deshpande, V., & Khosroshahi, A. (2012). Development of an IgG4-RD responder index. *International Journal of Rheumatology, 2012.* doi: 10.1155/2012/259408

Casian, A., & D'Cruz, D. (2016). Immunoglobulin G4 disease (IgG4-RD). Retrieved from http://www.vasculitis.org.uk/about-vasculitis/immunoglobulin-g4

de Buy Wenniger, L. J. M., Culver, E. L., & Beuers, U. (2014). Exposure to occupational antigens might predispose to IgG4-related disease. *Hepatology, 60*(4), 1453–1454.

Dodds, W. J. (1989). The physiology of swallowing. *Dysphagia, 3*(4), 171–178.

Hamano, H., Kawa, S., Horiuchi, A., Unno, H., Furuya, N., Akamatsu, T., . . . Kiyosawa, K. (2001). High serum IgG4 concentrations in patients with sclerosing pancreatitis. *New England Journal of Medicine, 344*(10), 732–738.

Inoue, D., Yoshida, K., Yoneda, N., Ozaki, K., Matsubara, T., Nagai, K., . . . Matsui, O. (2015). IgG4-related disease: Dataset of 235 consecutive patients. *Medicine, 94*(15).

Kamisawa, T., Zen, Y., Pillai, S., & Stone, J. H. (2015). IgG4-related disease. *The Lancet, 385*(9976), 1460–1471.

Karim, F., Loeffen, J., Bramer, W., Westenberg, L., Verdijk, R., van Hagen, M., & van Laar, J. (2016). IgG4-related disease: A systematic review of this unrecognized disease in pediatrics. *Pediatric Rheumatology Online Journal, 14*(1), 18. doi:10.1186/s12969-016-0079-3

Katsura, M., Morita, A., Horiuchi, H., Ohtomo, K., & Machida, T. (2011). IgG4-related inflammatory pseudotumor of the trigeminal nerve: Another component of IgG4-related sclerosing disease? *American Journal of Neuroradiology, 32*(8), E150–E152.

Khosroshahi, A., Wallace, Z. S., Crowe, J. L., Akamizu, T., Azumi, A., Carruthers, M. N., . . . Hart, P. A. (2015). International consensus guidance statement on the management and treatment of IgG4-related disease. *Arthritis & Rheumatology, 67*(7), 1688–1699.

Lopes, J., Hochwald, S. N., Lancia, N., Dixon, L. R., & Ben-David, K. (2010). Autoimmune esophagitis: IgG4-related tumors of the esophagus. *Journal of Gastrointestinal Surgery, 14*(6), 1031–1034.

Luiz, H. V., Gonçalves, D., Silva, T. N. D., Nascimento, I., Ribeiro, A., Mafra, M., . . . Portugal, J. (2014). IgG4-related Hashimoto's thyroiditis—A new variant of a well-known disease. *Arquivos Brasileiros de Endocrinologia & Metabologia, 58*(8), 862–868.

Nauntofte, B., & Jensen, J. L. (1999). Salivary secretion. In T. Yamada, D. H. Alpers, L. Laine, C. Owyang, & D. W. Powell (Eds). *Textbook of gastroenterology* (3rd ed., pp. 263–278). Philadelphia, PA: Lippencott Williams & Wilkins Publishers.

Obiorah, I., Hussain, A., Palese, C., Azumi, N., Benjamin, S., & Ozdemirli, M. (2017). IgG4-related disease involving the esophagus: A clinicopathological study. *Diseases of the Esophagus: Official Journal of the International Society for Diseases of the Esophagus, 30*(12), 1–7.

Oh, J. H., Lee, T. H., Kim, H. S., Jung, C. S., Lee, J. S., Hong, S. J., & Jin, S. Y. (2015). Esophageal involvement of immunoglobulin G4-related disease: A case report and literature review. *Medicine, 94*(50). doi: 10 .1097/MD.0000000000002122

Okazaki, K., & Umehara, H. (2012). Are classification criteria for IgG4-RD now possible? The concept of IgG4-related disease and proposal of comprehensive diagnostic criteria in Japan. *International Journal of Rheumatology, 2012*. doi: 10.1155/2012/357071

Pedersen, A. M., Bardow, A., Jensen, S. B., & Nauntofte, B. (2002). Saliva and gastrointestinal functions of taste, mastication, swallowing and digestion. *Oral Diseases, 8*(3), 117–129.

Pieringer, H., Parzer, I., Wöhrer, A., Reis, P., Oppl, B., & Zwerina, J. (2014). IgG4-related disease: An orphan disease with many faces. *Orphanet Journal of Rare Diseases, 9*(1), 110.

Shimizu, Y., Yamamoto, M., Naishiro, Y., Sudoh, G., Ishigami, K., Yajima, H., . . . Seki, N. (2012). Necessity of early intervention for IgG4-related disease—Delayed treatment induces fibrosis progression. *Rheumatology, 52*(4), 679–683.

Stone, J. H., Zen, Y., & Deshpande, V. (2012). IgG4-related disease. *New England Journal of Medicine, 366*(6), 539–551.

Wallace, Z. S., Carruthers, M. N., Khosroshahi, A., Carruthers, R., Shinagare, S., Stemmer-Rachamimov, A., . . . Stone, J. H. (2013). IgG4-related disease and hypertrophic pachymeningitis. *Medicine, 92*(4), 206.

Yoshida, K., Toki, F., Takeuchi, T., Watanabe, S. I., Shiratori, K., & Hayashi, N. (1995). Chronic pancreatitis caused by an autoimmune abnormality. *Digestive Diseases and Sciences, 40*(7), 1561–1568.

14

Esophageal Atresia

KEY WORDS: esophageal atresia, tracheoesophageal fistula, pharynx, cyanosis, VACTERL, Sequential Oral Sensory (SOS)

Definition

Esophageal atresia (EA) encompasses a group of rare, congenital malformations of the esophagus. In this rare, congenital defect, the infant is unable to pass food swallowed to the stomach. In most cases, the upper esophagus ends in a pouch that fails to connect with the lower esophagus and the stomach (Figure 14–1). EA is usually accompanied by a variety of congenital anatomic defects due to abnormal embryological development of the esophagus. For example, some infants with EA may have an accompanying condition called a **tracheoesophageal fistula** (TEF), which is an opening in the common wall that separates the trachea from the esophagus (Masahata et al., 2015). EA can also be considered as a malformation caused by the failure of the esophagus to develop as one continuous passage from the **pharynx** to the stomach during embryonic development. In the normal anatomy, the trachea connects to the lungs while the esophagus connects to the stomach. In EA, the esophagus fails to connect to the stomach

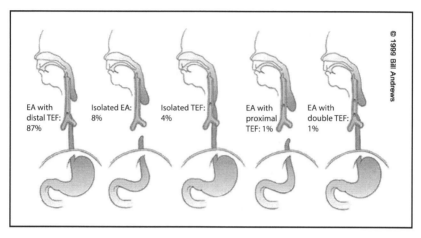

Figure 14–1. Types of esophageal atresia (EA) with and without tracheoesophageal fistula (TEF). *Source*: From "Esophageal Atresia and Tracheoesophageal Fistula," by D. C. Clark, 1999, *American Family Physician, 59*(4), 910–916.

during the development of the fetus, thus resulting in two segments: one part that connects to the pharynx and the other part to the stomach, but the segments are not connected to each other (Figure 14–1). Since the esophagus is now in two segments, liquids that the infant swallows cannot pass through the esophagus to the stomach. In the case of TEF, liquids swallowed by the infant can now enter the trachea and flow into the lungs, potentially causing aspiration pneumonia. Most infants with congenital forms of EA with TEF usually present shortly after birth with copious secretions, coughing, gagging, **cyanosis** (bluish discoloration of the skin due to inadequate oxygenation of the blood), vomiting, and respiratory distress.

The original classification of EA made by Vogt (1929) and modified by Gross (1953) continues to be used to this day. Gross' classification describes five types of esophageal atresia with accompanying TEF; these are categorized as types A through F (Figure 14–2).

Gross' type A is described as pure or isolated esophageal atresia without a fistula. In this type, the proximal and distal esoph-

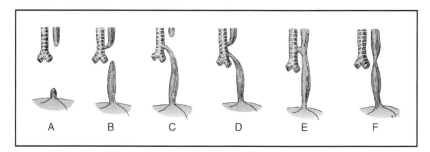

Figure 14–2. Gross' classification of EA. A = Pure esophageal atresia without fistula; B = Esophageal atresia with proximal tracheoesophageal fistula; C = Esophgeal atresia with distal tracheoesophageal fistula; D = Esophageal atresia with distal and proximal fistula; E = Tracheoesophageal fistula without atresia; F = Esophageal atresia/stenosis without fistula. *Source*: From "Anesthesia for General Surgery in the Neonate," by C. Brett and P. J. Davis, in P. J. Davis, F. P. Cladis, and E. K. Motoyama (Eds.), *Smith's Anesthesia for Infants and Children* (8th ed., pp. 554–588), 2011, Philadelphia, PA: Elsevier. Originally published in *The Surgery of Infancy and Childhood*, by R. E. Gross, 1953, Philadelphia, PA: W. B. Saunders.

agus end blindly without any connection to the trachea. Type B presents as an EA with proximal TEF. In this case, the fistula is sited on the proximal end of the upper pouch on the anterior wall of the esophagus. In type C, there is EA but with distal TEF. In type D, there is the presence of EA with proximal and distal TEF; whereas in type E, the anomaly presents as a TEF without EA. The frequency of occurrence of the various forms of EA varies. Type C appears to be the most common occurrence of EA with TEF, while Type D is the rarest form (Spitz, 2007) (Table 14–1).

EA with or without TEF is often associated with other anomalies. More than half of the infants with esophageal atresia present with one or more additional disorders such as **v**ertebral skeletal disorders, **a**norectal malformations, **c**ardiac disorders, **t**racheoesophageal fistula, **r**enal anomalies, and **l**imb deformities (**VACTERL**) (Sudjud, Bisri, & Boom, 2016). A concurrence of congenital anomalies not associated with a genetic disturbance is referred to as VACTERL, an acronym of the identified disorders noted above.

Table 14–1. Gross' Classification of EA and TEF, Description and Frequency

Type	Identification	Description	Frequency of Occurrence
A	Long gap/pure atresia	Gap between the two esophageal blind pouches with no fistula	7%
B	EA with proximal TEF	Upper esophageal pouch connected to trachea while lower esophageal pouch ends blindly	2%
C	EA with distal TEF	Lower esophageal pouch connects abnormally to trachea while upper esophageal pouch ends blindly	86%
D	EA with distal and proximal TEFs	Both upper and lower esophageal pouches join trachea in two different places	Less than 1%
E	TEF only, no EA (also known as H-type)	Normal intact esophagus, but an abnormal fistula/opening in the common wall	4%

Note: EA = esophageal atresia; TEF = tracheoesophageal fistula.

History

The first documented case of EA was made by Thomas Gibson more than 300 years ago in 1697, when he reported the case of an infant who was unable to swallow. The second recorded case was 150 years later by Thomas Hill, who described a newborn who was also unable to swallow (Spitz, 2007).

The first surgical attempts to repair EA were made by Lanman (1940), whose patients unfortunately did not survive. Early successes at EA repair were documented separately by Leven (1941) and Ladd (1944). Haight (1943), however, was credited with the first successful primary repair of the esophagus, performed in 1941. This monumental technical achievement formed the basis for the modern approach to surgery, and by the mid-1980s, successful surgery rates were more than 90%.

Etiology

The etiology of ER is largely unknown, but it is believed to be multifactorial. Research has shown embryological, genetic, and environmental factors may be implicated in the development of this disorder.

Embryological Factors

Although the mechanisms that undergird tracheoesophageal malformations are unclear, the reproduction in animal models of embryological anomalies has shed some light on the different stages of faulty **organogenesis**. In the study of embryology, organogenesis refers to the integrated processes that change cells into an organ in the developing embryo. By contrasting these stages in normal development, it is possible to pinpoint key developmental processes that may be disturbed during embryogenesis (Spitz, 2007).

The trachea, esophagus, and lungs are foregut-derived structures. During the fourth week of embryonic life, the foregut divides into a ventral respiratory portion that will eventually become the trachea/airway and a dorsal esophageal portion (de Jong, Felix, de Klein, & Tibboel, 2010). The underlying mechanism that gives rise to the separation is not known. One theory suggests that the trachea becomes a separate organ because of rapid longitudinal growth of the respiratory primordium away from the foregut (Merei, Hasthorpe, Farmer, & Hutson, 1998). A counter theory is that the trachea initially develops as a part of the undivided gut and then becomes a separate structure due to a separation process that begins at the level of the lung buds. This separate structure then continues to grow upward (Qi & Beasley, 2000). If there is an interruption in the normal process of separation, then the esophagus may become malformed, and thus lead to the development of EA with or without TEF.

Genetic Factors

According to Stoll, Alembik, Dott, and Roth (2009), greater than 50% of individuals with EA/TEF may exhibit some related anomaly. Some anomalies such as cardiovascular deficits, renal agenesis, microcephaly, duodenal atresia, and limb defects are prevalent in patients with EA/TEF. In many cases, EA/TEF may be present in several syndromes. In one notable syndrome, CHARGE (coloboma of the eye, heart defects, atresia of the choanae, retardation of growth, and ear abnormalities and deafness), about 10% of patients display EA/TEF. Some chromosomal aberrations have been reported in patients with EA/TEF. For example, individuals with Down syndrome and Edwards' syndrome may also exhibit EA/TEF. However, these may be co-occurrences and not causative.

Data from twin and family studies have shown to a lesser degree that the occurrence of more than one child with EA in a family is around 1%; moreover, the twin concordance rate is also low, about 2.5% (Shaw-Smith, 2006). This suggests that hereditary factors do not contribute largely to the etiology of EA. In fact, most cases of EA are sporadic, and the environmental risk factors seem to play a more essential role in the etiology of the disorder. Consequently, risk exposures of the pregnant mother during the early embryogenesis when the esophagus and the trachea are separating are particularly critical (Oddsberg, 2011). Ethnicity, drug use, tobacco smoking, alcohol use, and diabetes have all been identified as environmental risk factors for the development of EA/TEF.

Environmental Factors

Oddsberg, Jia, Nilsson, Ye, and Lagergren (2008) suggest an increased risk of having an infant with EA among white women compared to other ethnic groups. However, rather than pursue race as a factor, Oddsberg (2011) proposed that this proclivity may be more reflective of an interaction between environmental risk factors and genetic predispositions.

A few studies have examined the role of drugs in EA/TEF. A correspondence between the maternal use of drugs during early pregnancy and EA has been suggested by Lammer and Cordero (1986). Another potential link between maternal exposures to the medication methimazole for treatment of hyperthyroidism has been implicated as a causative factor in EA. Foulds, Walpole, Elmslie, and Mansour (2005) have reported several anomalies including gastrointestinal defects (such as EA) and dysmorphic facial features in infants exposed to carbimazole (medication for treatment of hyperthyroidism).

Combined use of tobacco smoking and alcohol use are well-documented factors in certain types of fetal defects. However, not many studies have specifically examined the link between maternal smoking and alcohol exposure and EA/TEF. One comprehensive study by Wong-Gibbons et al. (2008) failed to show a direct link, although other infant defects were identified.

Some associations between diabetes and EA have been reported in the literature. Based on a study of 2,625,436 newborn infants born to mothers with diabetes, 780 cases of EA were reported (Oddsberg, Lu, & Lagergren, 2010). These results strongly suggest that maternal diabetes can increase the infant's risk for EA. Other studies of insulin-dependent diabetic mothers suggest that exposure to maternal diabetes during the first trimester may be associated with EA/TEF as well as VACTERL-related anomalies (Castori, Rinaldi, Capocaccia, Roggini, & Grammatico, 2008).

Loane, Dolk, and Morris (2009) suggest that older mothers may be at significant risk of having a child with EA. On the other hand, Green et al. (2010) suggest that paternal age may be a risk factor for some multifactorial birth defects.

Epidemiology

The prevalence of rare abnormalities is established by global birth surveillance programs worldwide. Specifically, the prevalence of EA in Europe is reportedly stable, as reported by the National Birth Defects Prevention Network in the United States. In France, a reference center for congenital abnormalities of the esophagus was created in 2008. These various organizations have made it possible to establish epidemiological data (Sfeir, Michaud, Salleron & Gottrand, 2013). But the prevalence of EA is now known to vary across different geographical groups. The variation may also be reflected in the different presentations of EA (Table 14–2).

EA affects an average of 1 in 2,500 to 1 in 3,000 live births. The majority of EA cases appear to be sporadic, but even so, a small number of cases within this nonfamilial group appear to be associated with chromosomal abnormalities. Familial occurrences of EA are still considered rare, representing less than 1% of the total (Spitz, 2007).

In terms of gender and race, multiple studies have cautiously shown that EA is more common in males compared to females, and patients are more likely to be Caucasian than other racial or ethnic groups. However, most of these studies had many confounding variables such as age of diagnosis and the number of reported cases. For example, Sperry, Woosley, Shaheen, and Dellon (2012) found that Caucasians were older than African Americans at the time of diagnosis and males were more likely

Table 14–2. Associated Anomalies and Frequency of Occurrence in EA Globally

Country	Total Births	EA with TEF	EA without TEF	Total Cases	Prevalence Per 10,000 Births
Hungary	970,828	25	147	172	1.77
Georgia, USA	513,272	71	20	91	1.77
Texas, USA	3,305,512	495	102	597	1.81
Alberta, Canada	404,595	66	13	79	1.95
Slovak Republic	371,644	45	35	80	2.15
Paris, France	363,914	72	8	80	2.20
Saxony-Anhalt, Germany	162,723	24	14	38	2.34

Source: Adapted from "Prevalence of Esophageal Atresia Among 18 International Birth Defects Surveillance Programs," by N. Nassar, E. Leoncini, E. Amar, J. Arteaga-Vázquez, M. K. Bakker, C. Bower, . . . P. Mastroiacovo, 2012, *Birth Defects Research. Part A, Clinical and Molecular Teratology, 94*(11), 893–899. doi:10.1002/bdra.23067

to be diagnosed as children. Nevertheless, the symptoms of EA across all groups appear to be similar.

Clinical Presentation

Esophageal atresia is usually suspected early on in the prenatal ultrasound when a constellation of polyhydramnios (excess amniotic fluid in the amniotic sac), an absent or small fetal stomach bubble, and an upper pouch sign are present. Nevertheless, the first clinical signs of EA are clearly seen very soon after birth. The most common signs are frothy white bubbles in the mouth, excessive drooling, coughing, and gagging as well as intermittent cyanosis. Excessive oral secretions and drooling are characteristic of the newborn baby with EA. When suckling at the breast or bottle, the infant may have episodes of choking along with respiratory problems that may lead to cyanosis.

Most infants (more than 50%) with EA will present with one or multiple additional anomalies. Those systems that are affected tend to be cardiovascular, anorectal, genitourinary, gastrointestinal, vertebral/skeletal, and respiratory (de Jong et al., 2010).

Variations of EA/TEF tend to present with unique clinical manifestations of dysphagia (Table 14–3). For example, in EA with distal TEF—by far the most common type—the patient usually presents with significant coughing, regurgitation, excessive flow of saliva, and distention of the stomach. On the other hand, in atresia with proximal and distal fistulae—the rarest type—the patient may manifest excessive secretions and respiratory distress upon feeding.

Clinically, in the newborn infant with EA plus distal TEF (the most common form of EA), the lungs are constantly exposed to gastric secretions. Air from the trachea may pass down through the distal fistula to the stomach when the baby cries, strains, or breathes, thus leading to abdominal distention (Table 14–3). This causes severe feeding problems and ultimately leads to malnutrition if repair of the involved structures is delayed.

Table 14–3. Clinical Manifestations of Dysphagia in Different Types of EA/TEF

Type of EA/TEF	Clinical Manifestations	Diagnostic Findings	Management
EA with Distal TEF	Regurgitation, coughing, excessive saliva, stomach distention	Blind pouch	Surgical repair
EA without TEF	Excess oral secretions, regurgitation of feedings	Blind pouch without stomach distention	Two-step surgical process: (1) gastrostomy/cervical esophagostomy, (2) resection of esophagus
EA with Proximal TEF	Excessive oral secretions, respiratory distress with oral feedings	No abdominal air/distention	Surgery to repair esophagus and trachea
EA with Proximal and Distal TEF	Excessive oral secretions respiratory distress with oral feedings	Abdominal air	Surgery for ligation of the fistulae; esophagogastrostomy
TEF without EA/"H-Type"	Choking, coughing, distention of abdomen	Bronchoscopy to identify fistula	Surgery for ligation of the fistula

179

Since normal development of the trachea is impaired in EA, there can be structural weakening of the trachea leading to tracheomalacia. In this condition, the infant's cough is deep sounding, having the sonorous seal-bark quality with a choking or forceful exhalation. This results in difficulty clearing secretions, and places the infant at high risk for aspiration pneumonia.

Management of Dysphagia

Management of the infant with EA is usually medical–surgical, even though the treatment plan is individualized for each child. When EA is associated with TEF, it can be a life-threatening condition. This combination results in swallowing, digestion, and respiratory difficulties; thus, immediate medical and surgical interventions are warranted. In fact, the most important and effective treatment for EA/TEF is usually surgical. In many cases, the surgery is performed within 24 hours of birth. In other cases, depending on whether the infant has other complications such as infections or defects that would cause complications, the surgery may be delayed for a few months. Consequently, nutrition may be handled intravenously or by gastric feeding. In the latter case, the tube is inserted directly into the stomach.

Speech-Language Pathology Management

Lefton-Greif (2008) and Lefton-Greif et al. (2018), reported an increase in the occurrence of pediatric feeding and swallowing disorders. This may be due to the improved survival rate of infants with complex congenital disorders such as EA/TEF. This report urges the need for the speech-language pathologist (SLP)/ swallowing therapist to be trained in the appropriate management of swallowing disorders in this population.

The primary goals for infant feeding and swallowing disorders should be:

1. to provide safe and adequate nutrition and hydration

2. to provide the best methods and technique to maximize safe swallowing

3. to work with caregivers to incorporate diet preferences

4. to attain age appropriate eating skills

5. to minimize risks of aspiration

6. to maximize the person's quality of life

7. to create positive feeding experiences to the child (American Speech-Language-Hearing Association, 2019).

Children with EA/TEF require an interdisciplinary team approach for management of the dysphagia. This team is usually composed of disciplines appropriate for the specific case (Table 14–4), but the major provider on this team in many instances is the SLP/swallowing therapist who is trained in the area of dysphagia. However, the direct services of the SLP may not be required immediately, since the infant may still require tube feedings after the surgery.

There are common complications that occur secondary to EA/TEF repair of which the SLP should be aware. Some of these complications can be:

1. Esophageal dysmotility: this may occur because the esophageal wall musculature may be weakened.

2. Gastroesophageal reflux: most infants after EA/TEF repair tend to exhibit this condition. It is usually managed with medication.

3. TEF recurrence: this can only be managed surgically.

4. Chronic cough: this is a common symptom following esophageal atresia surgery because of the weakness of the trachea.

Table 14–4. Interdisciplinary Pediatric Feeding Team and Roles

Interdisciplinary Professional	Role/Function
Primary physician/pediatrician	Primary care of infant
Pediatric specialist: surgeon, neurologist, gastroenterologist, radiologist, pulmonologist, nurse practitioner	Diagnostic/medical care
Dietitian	Monitor child's overall nutritional requirements
Speech-language pathologist (SLP)	Swallowing assessment, diet safety, feeding techniques, caregiver education
Occupational therapist (OT)	Instruct and provide adaptive feeding equipment cotreatment with SLP, monitor motor/ sensory development
Physical therapist (PT)	Monitor sensory/motor development cotreatment with OT

The involvement of the SLP begins after all of the major medical issues have been resolved. Usually the main areas of concern are the child's oral motor skills, sensory integration skills, and physiological function. Since swallowing and feeding in the infant is so vital to life, the SLP has to be highly skilled in this area of caring for the infant. The next few sections will briefly touch on techniques/strategies that will be of interest to the SLP working with infants with feeding problems secondary to EA. Specifically, some essential considerations include the following:

1. The child's safety in feeding and swallowing.

2. The child's ability to obtain adequate nutrition by mouth alone.

3. The child's overall functional skills.

4. Behavioral or sensory–motor problems affecting the child's ability to eat or feed adequately.

The American Speech and Hearing Association (ASHA) suggests that the primary consideration of the SLP in treating pediatric dysphagia should be centered on the child's medical condition. This includes pulmonary integrity, nutritional status, and swallowing ability. These are critical issues as they can have serious ramifications on the safety of the swallow.

The SLP is responsible for working to help the infant achieve and maintain a safe swallow, as well as to ensure that the child who is being fed orally receives adequate nutrition. This determination is usually made in consultation with the dietitian. Consequently, recommendations as to whether the child should be fed orally or by an alternative method are critical decisions that the SLP will make. Factors that will inform these decisions are the length of time the child takes to feed/eat, the efficiency of the method of feeding, as well as whether fatigue is a major factor affecting the ability to be successful in eating.

In addition to determining the mode of feeding for the infant, the SLP also has to consider ways and means of maximizing the child's functional skills for safe feeding. To do this, careful assessment of the child's ability to orally manage the least restrictive type of consistency with or without compensatory strategies.

One other area that must be considered in managing dysphagia secondary to EA is the child's response to the whole idea of feeding. It is not infrequent that many children have an aversion to oral feeding after surgical repair of the EA. This may be due to the lack of experience with oral feeding since the infant may have been on tube feedings presurgery. In this case, management of feeding may take the form of creating an environment in which the child can derive a sense of pleasure from the eating experience.

To date, no single approach or method has been identified as the most effective in helping the child to feed and swallow after the repair of the esophagus in EA. However, factors that must be considered in the management process are the child's perspective, the parent/caregiver, the child's medical history, and the duration of the treatment. One approach described by Toomey (2000) that is frequently used with infants from birth to 18 years is the **Sequential Oral Sensory (SOS)** feeding program. This treatment approach helps the postsurgery child to develop an affinity for oral feeding through integrating posture, motor learning, medical, and nutritional factors (Toomey, 2000). The child learns to interact with the food by first tolerating the very presence of the food, touching it, and eventually tasting the food. This approach suggests the importance of the therapist and the caregiver paying attention to the infant's cues during feeding.

Crary and Groher (2016) described the principles of cue-based care/developmentally supportive care in feeding infants with swallowing problems. In bottle feeding, both the equipment—such as the bottle and the nipple—used as well as the actions of the feeder can negatively or positively impact the infant's performance in feeding.

The principles of *cue-based care (CBC)* emphasize that those who care for the infant should observe and respond appropriately "to the infant's cues" during all caregiving tasks including feeding. Some principles of CBC suggest that the infant should be at optimum arousal and physiological stability before presentation of the bottle. Being attentive to the unique needs of the infant learning to accept oral feedings is critical for successful transition from tube feedings to oral feedings.

Summary

Esophageal atresia or EA is a rare, congenital disorder of the digestive tract. It results from a separation of the upper esophagus from the lower portion that leads to the stomach. It is usually found in combination with a tracheoesophageal fistula. It can be diagnosed as early as during the antenatal period or shortly after birth.

The incidence of EA is estimated to be around 1 in 2,500 to 1 in 4,500 live births. These numbers may vary depending on location. Esophageal atresia tends to be a sporadic occurrence in families; consequently, there is a very low likelihood of the disorder recurring in siblings.

The etiology of EA or EA/TEF to date is unclear. However, it is often associated with some genetic syndromes such as Down syndrome, CHARGE syndrome, and Edwards' syndrome. However, EA tends to occur more often with the VACTERL anomalies. Esophageal atresia with tracheoesophageal malformations occur as a spectrum of anomalies. Many classifications have been made of these forms. The most common classification is referred to as Gross' classification. In this scheme, five types of EA/TEF have been identified: Types A, B, C, D, and E. Type A is described as EA without TEF, type B is EA with proximal TEF, type C is EA with distal TEF, type D is EA with proximal and distal TEF, and type E is TEF without EA.

Clinically, babies with EA and TEF present postnatally with the inability to handle their own saliva. It is very common for them to display coughing, choking, and swallowing difficulties. Management is always surgical. The SLP is mostly involved in the treatment when the infant or child is learning or relearning how to feed orally.

References

American Speech-Language-Hearing Association [ASHA]. (n.d.). *Pediatric dysphagia*. Retrieved 28 July 2019 from https://www.asha.org /Practice-Portal/Clinical-Topics/Pediatric-Dysphagia/

Brett, C., & Davis, P. J. (2011). Anesthesia for general surgery in the neonate. In P. J. Davis, F. P. Cladis, & E. K. Motoyama (Eds.), *Smith's anesthesia for infants and children* (8th ed., pp. 554–588). Philadelphia, PA: Elsevier.

Castori, M., Rinaldi, R., Capocaccia, P., Roggini, M., & Grammatico, P. (2008). VACTERL association and maternal diabetes: A possible causal relationship? *Birth Defects Research Part A: Clinical and Molecular Teratology, 82*(3), 169–172.

Clark, D. C. (1999). Esophageal atresia and tracheoesophageal fistula. *American Family Physician, 59*(4), 910–916.

Crary, M. A., & Groher, M. E. (2016). *Dysphagia: Clinical management in adults and children.* St. Louis, MO: Elsevier Health Sciences.

de Jong, E. M., Felix, J. F., de Klein, A., & Tibboel, D. (2010). Etiology of esophageal atresia and tracheoesophageal fistula: "Mind the gap." *Current Gastroenterology Reports, 12*(3), 215–222.

Foulds, N., Walpole, I., Elmslie, F., & Mansour, S. (2005). Carbimazole embryopathy: An emerging phenotype. *American Journal of Medical Genetics Part A, 132*(2), 130–135.

Green, R. F., Devine, O., Crider, K. S., Olney, R. S., Archer, N., Olshan, A. F., . . . Study, T. N. B. D. P. (2010). Association of paternal age and risk for major congenital anomalies from the National Birth Defects Prevention Study, 1997 to 2004. *Annals of Epidemiology, 20*(3), 241–249.

Gross, R. E. (1953). The surgery of infancy and childhood. *Omental cysts and mesentric cysts* (pp. 377–383), Philadelphia, PA: Saunders.

Haight, C. (1943). Congenital atresia of the esophagus with traceoesophageal fistula. *Surgery, Gynecology, and Obstetrics, 76,* 672–676.

Ladd, W. E. (1944). The surgical treatment of esophageal atresia and tracheoesophageal fistulas. *New England Journal of Medicine, 230*(21), 625–637.

Lammer, E. J., & Cordero, J. F. (1986). Exogenous sex hormone exposure and the risk for major malformations. *JAMA, 255*(22), 3128–3132.

Lanman, T. H. (1940). Congenital atresia of the esophagus: A study of thirty-two cases. *Archives of Surgery, 41*(5), 1060–1083.

Lefton-Greif, M. A. (2008). Pediatric dysphagia. *Physical Medicine and Rehabilitation Clinics, 19*(4), 837–851.

Lefton-Greif, M. A., McGrattan, K. E., Carson, K. A., Pinto, J. M., Wright, J. M., & Martin-Harris, B. (2018). First steps towards development of an instrument for the reproducible quantification of oropharyngeal swallow physiology in bottle-fed children. *Dysphagia, 33*(1), 76–82.

Leven, N. L. (1941). Congenital atresia of esophagus with tracheoesophageal fistula. *Journal of Thoracic and Cardiovascular Surgery, 10,* 648–657.

Loane, M., Dolk, H., & Morris, J. K. (2009). Maternal age-specific risk of non-chromosomal anomalies. *BJOG: An International Journal of Obstetrics & Gynaecology, 116*(8), 1111–1119.

Masahata, K., Hasegawa, T., Kuroda, S., Takahashi, N., Nojima, I., Kimura, N., . . . Kubota, A. (2015). A rare variant case of pure esophageal atresia with an atretic segment. *Journal of Pediatric Surgery Case Reports, 3*(9), 389–391.

Merei, J. M., Hasthorpe, S., Farmer, P., & Hutson, J. M. (1998). Embryogenesis of tracheal atresia. *The Anatomical Record: An Official Publication of the American Association of Anatomists, 252*(2), 271–275.

Oddsberg, J. (2011). Environmental factors in the etiology of esophageal atresia. *Journal of Pediatric Gastroenterology and Nutrition, 52*, S4–S5.

Oddsberg, J., Jia, C., Nilsson, E., Ye, W., & Lagergren, J. (2008). Influence of maternal parity, age, and ethnicity on risk of esophageal atresia in the infant in a population-based study. *Journal of Pediatric Surgery, 43*(9), 1660–1665.

Oddsberg, J., Lu, Y., & Lagergren, J. (2010). Maternal diabetes and risk of esophageal atresia. *Journal of Pediatric Surgery, 45*(10), 2004–2008.

Qi, B. Q., & Beasley, S. W. (2000). Stages of normal tracheo-bronchial development in rat embryos: Resolution of a controversy. *Development, Growth & Differentiation, 42*(2), 145–153.

Sfeir, R., Michaud, L., Salleron, J., & Gottrand, F. (2013). Epidemiology of esophageal atresia. *Diseases of the Esophagus, 26*(4), 354–355.

Shaw-Smith, C. (2006). Oesophageal atresia, tracheo-oesophageal fistula, and the VACTERL association: Review of genetics and epidemiology. *Journal of Medical Genetics, 43*(7), 545–554.

Sperry, S. L., Woosley, J. T., Shaheen, N. J., & Dellon, E. S. (2012). Influence of race and gender on the presentation of eosinophilic esophagitis. *American Journal of Gastroenterology, 107*(2), 215.

Spitz, L. (2007). Oesophageal atresia. *Orphanet Journal of Rare Diseases, 2*(1), 24.

Stoll, C., Alembik, Y., Dott, B., & Roth, M. P. (2009). Associated malformations in patients with esophageal atresia. *European Journal of Medical Genetics, 52*(5), 287–290.

Sudjud, R., Bisri, T., & Boom, C. E. (2016). Anesthetic consideration on neonatal patient with esophageal atresia. *Open Journal of Anesthesiology, 6*(9), 128.

Toomey, K. A. (2000). *Picky eaters versus problem feeders* [PDF]. Retrieved from https://www.spdstar.org/sites/default/files/file-attachments/Picky%20Eaters%20vs%20Problem%20Feeders_1.pdf

Vogt, E. C. (1929). Congenital esophageal atresia. *American Journal of Roentgenology, 22*(463–464), 465.

Wong-Gibbons, D. L., Romitti, P. A., Sun, L., Moore, C. A., Reefhuis, J., Bell, E. M., & Olshan, A. F. (2008). Maternal periconceptional exposure to cigarette smoking and alcohol and esophageal atresia±tracheoesophageal fistula. *Birth Defects Research Part A: Clinical and Molecular Teratology, 82*(11), 776–784.

15

Wallenberg Syndrome

KEY WORDS: Wallenberg syndrome, cerebellar artery, lateral medullary syndrome, Horner's syndrome, anhidrosis, ptosis

Definition

Wallenberg syndrome (WS) is a rare neurological condition caused by a stroke in the posterior inferior **cerebellar artery** of the brain stem. WS is also known as lateral medullary syndrome because it occurs in the part of the brain stem known as the lateral medulla. The nuclei of cranial nerves IX (the glossopharyngeal) and X (the vagus) appear to be involved in this disorder. The actual cause of the syndrome is relatively unclear.

History

The earliest description of WS was described in the case study of Gaspard Vieusseux of Geneva in London. Marcet (1811) described a case of vertigo, unilateral facial numbness, dysphagia, and drooped eyelids. However, several years later, Adolf Wallenberg

(1895) accurately identified the site of lesion and the symptoms of the disorder with his name bearing the eponym "Wallenberg syndrome."

Wallenberg published several reports on the disorder. In his seminal publication, he described a 38-year-old male with symptoms such as vertigo, hyperesthesia of the left side of his face and body, and dysphagia with impaired sensation of the mucosa of the mouth, throat, and palate. After the death of this patient, Wallenberg was able to substantiate his clinical findings upon postmortem examination of the patient. It is interesting to note that the symptoms Wallenberg described so many years ago continue to be the set of symptoms that are characteristic of WS to date.

Etiology

The most common underlying cause of WS is a brain stem stroke within the posterior inferior arteries of the brain stem (Figure 15–1). However, several other conditions have been suggested as causal links to WS. Some of these include trauma to the vertebral artery in the neck, metastatic cancer, aneurysm of the vertebral artery, head injury, arteriovenous malformations (AVMs), multiple sclerosis, and infections.

The most common risk factors for WS are hypertension and collagen vascular disease (Lui, Tadi, & Anilkumar, 2019). According to Field and Barton (2010), lateral medullary strokes, another term for WS, comprise about 2% of ischemic infarcts in the territory of the posterior inferior cerebellar artery (PICA), while 75% to 90% of large vessel **lateral medullary syndrome** is due to vertebral artery disease, with the remaining due to sporadic PICA infarcts. In a review of 130 cases of WS, these authors found 50% of the cases to be attributed to large vessel diseases, with the remainder distributed as dissection (15%), small vessel disease (13%), embolism due to cardiac problems (5%), and unknown causes (15%).

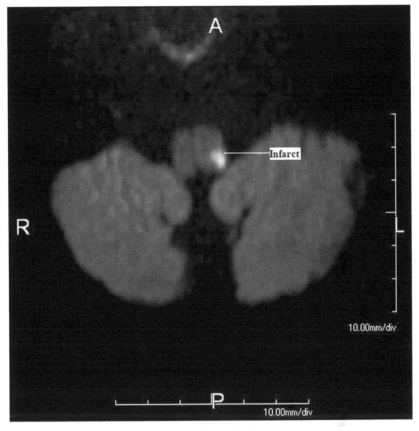

Figure 15–1. Left dorsal lateral infarct causing WS. *Source*: From John S. To (https://commons.wikimedia.org/wiki/File:WallenbergInfarct001.jpg), "Wallen-bergInfarct001," marked as public domain.

Epidemiology

WS appears to affect more males than females and the onset is typically in late adulthood. Various studies have confirmed this finding. Sacco, Freddo, Bello, Odel, Onesti, and Mohr (1993) studied 33 patients with WS and noted that their ages ranged from 24 to 83 years of age. Furthermore, 23 of the 33 patients were males. Studies carried out in Australia by Aydogdu, Ertekin, Tarlaci, Turman, Kiylioglu, and Secil (2001) found that in a group of 20 patients, the ages ranged from 37 to 75 years and there were 17 males and 3 female. WS is rarely seen in children—to date, there have only been five reported cases.

Clinical Presentation

The specific clinical manifestations of WS are largely determined by the location of the lesion in the brain stem. For example, the nucleus ambiguus is a group of large motor neurons located deep in the medullary reticular formation. These contain the cell bodies of nerves that innervate the muscles of the soft palate, pharynx, and larynx—structures that are highly associated with speech and swallowing. If the lesion is specifically in the nucleus ambiguus, the major clinical symptoms will be dysphagia, dysarthria, and dysphonia.

In WS, there is a constellation of neurological symptoms secondary to the lateral medullary involvement. These are sensory deficits affecting the torso and extremities on the contralateral side of the infarct. Typically, a person who presents with WS may exhibit varied symptoms depending on the locus of the lesion (Table 15–1). However, the most common symptoms of WS are dysphagia, dysarthria, ataxia, facial numbness that may also involve the body, and **Horner's syndrome**. Horner's syndrome is a condition in which there is a disruption of the nerve pathway from the brain to the face and eye (sympathetic nerve) unilaterally. The individual usually exhibits miosis (small pupil) compared to the unaffected eye, reduced dilation of the affected pupil in dim light, **ptosis** (drooping of the upper eyelid), and reduced sweating on the one side of the face (**anhidrosis**).

Table 15–1. Site of Lesion and Accompanying Deficits

Site of Lesions	Clinical Symptoms
Spinothalamic tract, descending nucleus, and tract of cranial nerve V	Loss of pain and temperature sensation on contralateral and ipsilateral sides
Nucleus ambiguus, and efferent fibers of CN IX and CN X	Dysphagia, dysphonia, dysarthria, laryngeal, and pharyngeal and palatal paralysis
Trigeminal nucleus	Numbness of the contralateral face as well as ipsilateral facial and corneal anesthesia
Hypothalamic fibers, descending sympathetic tract	Horner's syndrome
Deiter's nucleus and other vestibular nuclei	Nystagmus and vertigo
Central tegmental tract	Palatal myoclonus
Cerebellum	Ataxia

Dysphagia in WS

Swallowing is a complex motor event. Central control of swallowing is regulated by a central pattern generator (CPG), which is located in the solitary tract nucleus in the reticular formation of the medulla (Figure 15–2). Swallowing takes place when the CPG activates the motor neurons of the cranial nerve. The nucleus ambiguus as well as the vagal dorsal motor nucleus are also activated; these all act to innervate the muscles that are involved in swallowing (Martino, Terrault, Ezerzer, Mikulis, & Diamant, 2001). From a physiological perspective, if the CPG in the brain stem fails to program the entire pharyngeal swallow to trigger, the bolus will simply fall into the pyriform sinuses or into the airway. This is usually the case in WS. Specific swallowing difficulties

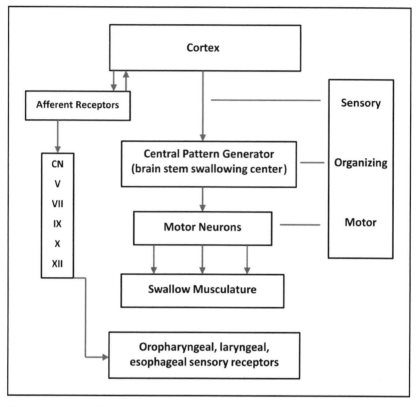

Figure 15–2. Swallowing center of the brain stem (central pattern generator). *Source*: From *Dysphagia evaluation and treatment*, by E. Saitoh, K. Pongpipatpaiboon, Y. Inamoto, and H. Kagaya, 2018, Gateway East, Singapore: Springer Singapore.

occur when there is an infarct in the swallowing centers of the rostral dorsolateral medulla, as in the case of a lateral medullary infarction (LMI), resulting in the classic swallowing symptoms unique to WS.

From a neurological perspective, there appears to be a single mechanism that underlies bilateral medullary swallowing centers, causing them to function as one integrated center. Consequently, an infarct to a portion of the swallowing center is sufficient to render a complete dissolution of the ability to swallow (Vigderman, Chavin, Kososky, & Tahmoush, 1998). Dysphagia secondary to WS tends to be more severe compared to dysphagia due to cortical strokes. In WS, dysphagia is frequently the outstanding deficit and it lasts longer compared to that of individuals with cortical strokes. Additionally, the dysphagia in WS is much more severe in comparison to that seen in cortical strokes. Consequently, most WS patients may require alternative feeding initially, but recovery in some cases is seen in less than three months. In this author's experience, recovery in which the patient was able to eat controlled amounts of pureed foods was typically seen around twelve months in the few patients treated.

Dysphagia in WS is usually associated with pharyngeal phase deficits as well as dysfunction of the upper esophageal sphincter (UES). During the swallowing, there is contraction of the proximal pharynx and an absence of motor activity in both the UES and the proximal esophagus. In this condition, visualization of the swallow during videofluoroscopy will often reveal material stuck at the level of the UES and throughout the pharyngeal area.

Management of Dysphagia

As previously stated, many patients with WS will require alternative feeding such as a PEG tube. However, there are technological advances such as VitalStim therapy, transcranial magnetic stimulation (TMS), and functional magnetic stimulation (FMS) that have significantly improved the assessment and management of dysphagia in patients with WS (Gupta & Banerjee, 2014). Traditional therapy such as the Mendelsohn maneuver has proven successful; however, both patient and clinician must be willing to invest time and effort in order to achieve success. There have been many cases clinically reported by this author in which patients have been able to return to a regular diet following a course of systematic therapy utilizing the Mendelsohn maneuver as an indirect treatment protocol while the patient received PEG tube feedings (Figure 15–3). A sample case report is provided in Figure 15–4.

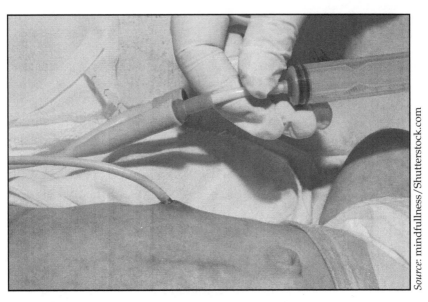

Figure 15–3. Percutaneous endoscopic gastrostomy (PEG).

R was a 55-year-old male who suffered a lateral medullary infarct. R was ambulatory post stroke, but exhibited a hoarse vocal quality with moderate dysarthria. He reported difficulty swallowing. On first encounter with R, he was noted with difficulty swallowing his oral secretions and consequently, required frequent oral suctioning. MBS performed revealed pharyngeal dysphagia characterized by reduced pharyngeal contraction resulting in pooling in the valleculae and pyriforms. There was absent relaxation of the UES. Overt aspiration occurred from the pooled material in the pyriforms. The residue of material had to be suctioned from the pharyngeal area.

Management: R received a naso-gastric feeding tube initially, but two weeks later, he was given a percutaneous endoscopic gastrostomy (PEG) as it was unlikely that his oral feeding would improve substantially within the ensuing several weeks. He was seen by the speech-language pathologist who provided a strict regimen of laryngeal tasks as well as the Mendelsohn maneuver after four weeks of exercises, a repeat MBS showed that R was able to swallow small sips of liquids including ice chips. This heightened his level of motivation. He continued receiving therapy with the SLP and in three months, R was able to swallow applesauce. Within one year, R was able to tolerate pureed foods and thin liquids. He continued to improve until eventually he was able to tolerate soft solids and thin liquids. His PEG was eventually removed, and R was advanced to an oral diet.

Figure 15–4. Case report.

It is noteworthy that among the many symptoms present in WS, those that bear significance for swallowing include dysarthria, hoarseness, and dysphonia. According to Groher (1992), reported vocal fold paralysis is common, and this leads to aspiration as well as a weak cough. Aydogdu et al. (2001) found that 85% of their patients with dysphagia secondary to WS exhibited vocal fold paresis and a weak cough. Earlier studies by Horner, Massey, Riski, Lathrop, and Chase (1988) reported more than 93% of their WS patients with dysphagia also presented with dysphonia.

Summary

WS is a condition that affects the nervous system. Signs and symptoms may include swallowing difficulties, dizziness, hoarseness, nausea and vomiting, nystagmus, and problems with balance. Wallenberg syndrome is often caused by trauma or an infarct in the posterior lateral medullary area. For reasons not very clearly understood, the condition appears to be present in more males than females. Treatment approach is more effective from a multidisciplinary perspective to address the myriad symptoms that are present.

Dysphagia is one of the primary symptoms. Treatment for this condition often includes a feeding tube for swallowing problems, speech and/or swallowing therapy, and medication for pain. While some individuals' symptoms may improve within months, others may have long-term neurological problems.

References

Aydogdu, I., Ertekin, C., Tarlaci, S., Turman, B., Kiylioglu, N., & Secil, Y. (2001). Dysphagia in lateral medullary infarction (Wallenberg's syndrome): An acute disconnection syndrome in premotor neurons related to swallowing activity? *Stroke, 32*(9), 2081–2087.

Field, T., & Barton, J. (2010). *Prenuclear disorders: Brainstem.* Retrieved 30 July, 2019, from http://www.neuroophthalmology.ca/textbook /disorders-of-eye-movements/v-prenuclear-disorders-brainstem/i -wallenbergs-lateral-medullary-syndrome

Groher, M. E. (1992). Establishing a swallowing program. In M. E. Groher (Ed.), *Dysphagia, diagnosis and management* (2nd ed., pp. 313–325). Boston, MA: Butterworth-Heinemann.

Homer, J., Massey, E. W., Riski, J. E., Lathrop, D. L., & Chase, K. N. (1988). Aspiration following stroke: Clinical correlates and outcome. *Neurology, 38*(9), 1359–1359.

Lui, F., Tadi, P., & Anilkumar A. C. (2019). *Wallenberg syndrome.* Retrieved from https://www.ncbi.n1m.nih.gov/books/NBK470174/

Marcet, A. (1811). History of a singular nervous or paralytic affection attended with anomalous morbid sensations. *Medico-Chirurgical Transactions, 2*, 215–233.

Martino, R., Terrault, N., Ezerzer, F., Mikulis, D., & Diamant, N. E. (2001). Dysphagia in a patient with lateral medullary syndrome: Insight into the central control of swallowing. *Gastroenterology, 121*(2), 420–426.

Sacco, R. L., Freddo, L., Bello, J. A., Odel, J. G., Onesti, S. T., & Mohr, J. P. (1993). Wallenberg's lateral medullary syndrome: Clinical-magnetic resonance imaging correlations. *Archives of Neurology, 50*(6), 609–614.

Saitoh, E., Pongpipatpaiboon, K., Inamoto, Y., & Kagaya, H. (2018). *Dysphagia evaluation and treatment.* Gateway East, Singapore: Springer Singapore.

Vigderman, A. M., Chavin, J. M., Kososky, C., & Tahmoush, A. J. (1998). Aphagia due to pharyngeal constrictor paresis from acute lateral medullary infarction. *Journal of the Neurological Sciences, 155*(2), 208–210.

Wallenberg, A. (1895). Acute bulbäraffection (embolism of the species cerebellar, post inf. Sinistr). *European Archives of Psychiatry and Clinical Neuroscience, 27*(2), 504–540.

Glossary

Achalasia: A rare disease of the muscle of the lower esophageal body and the lower esophageal sphincter that prevents relaxation of the sphincter and an absence of contractions, or peristalsis, of the esophagus.

Acid sphingomyelinase: An enzyme from the sphingomyelinase family, responsible for catalyzing the breakdown of sphingomyelin to ceramide and phosphorylcholine.

Alglucosidase alfa: An enzyme replacement therapy (ERT) orphan drug for treating Pompe disease.

Angular cheilitis: Inflammation of one or both corners of the mouth, characterized by erythema, cracked lips, bleeding, and ulcerated corners of the lips.

Anhidrosis: The inability to sweat normally; also known as hypohidrosis.

Antigen: Any substance that can stimulate the production of antibodies.

Apraxia: A motor disorder caused by damage to the posterior parietal cortex of the brain in which the individual has difficulty with the motor planning to perform tasks or movements when asked.

Aspiration: The passage of material past the vocal folds and into the trachea.

Aspiration pneumonia: A complication of pulmonary aspiration in which material is inhaled into the trachea.

Ataxia: Poor coordination of motor functioning or lack of order of muscle movements.

Ataxia telangiectasia: A rare, progressive, monogenic neurodegenerative disease with a pattern of autosomal recessive inheritance; also known as Louis-Bar syndrome. This disorder is characterized by ataxia, immunodeficiency, sino-pulmonary infections, premature aging, nutritional compromise, and dysphagia.

Atresia: Absence or abnormal narrowing of an opening or passage in the body.

Atrophy: A decrease in size or a wasting away of a body part or tissue.

Autoantigen: An antigen of one's own cells or cell products.

Autosomal recessive: A mode of inheritance of a trait or disorder that is passed from one generation to another. If both parents are carriers, there is a 25% chance of an offspring inheriting both abnormal genes and thus developing the disease. There is a 50% chance of a child inheriting only one abnormal gene and becoming a carrier (just as the parents), and, alternatively, there is a 25% chance of a child inheriting both normal genes.

Autosomes: Any chromosome that is not a sex chromosome.

Biotin-thiamine-responsive basal ganglia disease (BTBGD): A rare, autosomal recessive neurometabolic disorder characterized by subacute encephalopathy, confusion, seizures, dysarthria, dysphagia, and dystonia.

Botulinum toxin: A toxin produced by the bacterium *Clostridium botulinum*. This is the most poisonous biological substance known.

Bronchopulmonary dysplasia: A form of chronic lung disease that affects newborns and infants, resulting from damage to the lungs caused by mechanical ventilation and long-term use of oxygen.

Camptodactyly: Permanent flexion of one or more finger joints.

Cataplexy: Debilitating condition in which a person suddenly feels weak, especially during a time of strong emotion; for example, anger, fear, or surprise.

Ceramide: Lipids that help form the skin's barrier and retain skin's moisture.

Cerebellar artery: An artery that provides blood to the cerebellum.

Cerebellar ataxia: Incoordination of movements because of lesions in the afferent and efferent cerebellar connections.

Chromosomes: A threadlike structure of nucleic acids and proteins found in the nucleus of most living cells, carrying genetic information in the form of genes.

Congenital: Of a disease or physical abnormality; present from birth.

Congenital esophageal stenosis: A rare anomaly due to incomplete separation of the primitive foregut from the respiratory tract around the 25th week of life.

Consanguineous: Relating to or denoting people descended from the same ancestor.

Corneal reflex: Involuntary blinking of the eyelids.

Cyanosis: Bluish discoloration of the skin due to inadequate oxygenation of the blood.

Diaphragmatic myopathy: A decrease in the strength of the diaphragm.

Dilatation: Stretching of a tube or orifice beyond normal dimensions by either medication or instrumentation.

Diplegia: Paralysis of corresponding parts on both sides of the body, typically affecting the legs more severely than the arms.

Dwarfism: Unusually or abnormally low stature.

Dysarthria: A group of motor speech disorders resulting from neurological injury to the motor component of the motor-speech system.

Dysautonomia: Abnormal functioning of the autonomic nervous system.

Dyskinesia: Impairment of voluntary muscle movements resulting in fragmented or jerky movements.

Dysmorphism: An anatomical malformation.

Dysphagia: A medical term used to describe difficulty swallowing and encompassing four primary phases: oral preparatory (mastication), oral, pharyngeal, and esophageal.

Dysphonia: Involuntary spasms in the muscles of the larynx.

Dysplasia: Abnormal development or growth of cells, organs, or tissues.

Dystonia: A movement disorder in which a person's muscles contract uncontrollably, and may affect one muscle, a muscle group, or the entire body.

Encephalopathy: A term that means brain disease, damage, or malfunction, characterized by memory loss, personality changes, seizures, coma, and dementia.

Epidemiology: The branch of medicine which deals with the incidence, distribution, and possible control of diseases and other factors relating to health.

Erythema: Superficial reddening of the skin, usually in patches, as a result of injury or irritation causing dilatation of the blood capillaries.

Esophageal atresia: A congenital defect in which the upper esophagus does not connect with the lower esophagus.

Esophageal strictures: A narrowing or tightening of the esophagus; also known as a stenosis.

Esophageal web: A congenital or acquired transverse fold of mucous membrane that is found in the layers of the esophagus causing dysphagia.

Esophagus: A muscular tube connecting the pharynx with the stomach, lined with mucosa, providing a pathway for material to the stomach.

Etiology: The cause, set of causes, or manner of causation of a disease or condition.

Fahr's disease: A rare, genetically dominant, neurological disorder characterized by abnormal deposits of calcium in areas of the brain such as the basal ganglia, thalamus, hippocampus, and cerebral cortex. Symptoms include progressive deterioration of motor function, declining intellect, seizures, motor speech disorders, spasticity, visual impairments, dysphagia, dystonia, psychiatric disturbances, and parkinsonism.

Fistula: An abnormal or surgically made passage between a hollow or tubular organ and the body surface, or between two hollow or tubular organs.

Gastroesophageal reflux disease (GERD): A condition in which stomach acid frequently flows back into the esophagus because the muscle at the lower esophagus, known as the lower esophageal sphincter (LES), fails to close properly. This causes the contents of the stomach to leak back (reflux) into the esophagus, thus irritating it.

Gastrostomy (GT) tube: A tube inserted through the abdomen that delivers nutrition to the directly stomach.

Genotype: The genetic composition of an organism with respect to a single or multiple traits.

Glossitis: A general term for inflammation of the tongue, often characterized by depapillation of the dorsal aspects of the tongue.

Hepatosplenomegaly: A medical condition in which the liver and the spleen become enlarged.

Horner's syndrome: A condition in which there is a disruption of the nerve pathway from the brain to the face and eye unilaterally, characterized by miosis compared to the unaffected eye, reduced dilation of the affected pupil in dim light, ptosis, and anhidrosis.

Hypercarbia: Abnormally elevated carbon dioxide levels in the blood.

Hypertelorism: Abnormally increased distance between two organs or body parts, usually referring to an increased distance between the eyes.

Hyperthermia: Abnormally increased body temperature.

Hypertonicity: A condition in which muscle tone is abnormally tight or taut.

Hypoplasia: Incomplete development or underdevelopment of an organ or tissue.

Hypotonia: A state of low muscle tone, often involving reduced muscle strength; also known as "floppy baby syndrome."

Immunodeficiency: A state in which the immune system's ability to fight infectious disease and cancer is compromised or entirely absent.

Immunoglobulin G4-related disease: A group of immune-mediated diseases with common clinical, serological, and pathological features.

Iron deficiency anemia: A common type of anemia in which blood lacks adequate healthy red blood cells due to decreased levels of iron.

Koilonychia: A condition in which the fingernails present as thin with lifted outer edges, resembling the shape of a spoon, caused by iron deficiency or poor absorption of iron.

Laryngeal webbing: A rare condition in which the trachea is partially constricted by a weblike tissue that limits the volume of air flowing in and out of the larynx.

Larynx: The hollow muscular organ forming an air passage to the lungs and holding the vocal cords; it is made up of 9 total cartilages:

3 unpaired (epiglottis, thyroid, cricoid) and 3 paired (arytenoids, cuneiforms, corniculates).

Lateral medullary syndrome: *See* Wallenberg syndrome.

Leukemia inhibiting factor receptor (LIFR) gene: A specific gene that provides instruction for making the LIFR. The receptor spans the cell membrane thus allowing it to bind to other proteins.

Louis-Bar syndrome: *See* ataxia telangiectasia.

Lumen: The inside space of a tubular structure.

Lysosomes: Membrane-bound compartments (organelles) present in eukaryotic cells that are responsible for digesting and recycling molecules.

Macroglossia: The abnormal enlargement of the tongue.

Malformation: A deformity; an abnormally formed part of the body.

Mendelsohn maneuver: Voluntary prolongation of hyolaryngeal elevation at the peak of the swallow.

Microcephaly: Abnormally small head, usually associated with neuro-developmental delay.

Microstomia: Abnormal smallness of the mouth.

Miosis: Excessive constriction of the pupil of the eye.

Moebius syndrome: A rare neurological condition that primarily affects the muscles that control facial expression and eye movement, characterized by weakness or paralysis of the facial muscles.

Mutation: A permanent alteration in the DNA sequence that makes up a gene such that the sequence differs from what is found in most people; the alteration can range in size, affecting anywhere from a single DNA base pair to a large segment of a chromosome that involves multiple genes.

Myopathy: A disease of the muscle tissue.

Myositis: Inflammation and degeneration of muscle tissue.

Nasogastric tube: A medically placed tube that carries food and medicine to the stomach through the nose.

Nemaline myopathy: A congenital, autosomal recessive, hereditary neuromuscular disorder characterized by respiratory deficiency, delayed motor development, and muscle weakness that is more pronounced in proximal muscles as opposed to more distal muscles.

Niemann-Pick disease: An autosomal recessive disorder in the group of lysosomal storage diseases that interferes with metabolism.

Nocturnal hypoventilation: A condition in which there is poor breathing during sleep that results in increased levels of carbon dioxide in the blood.

NORD: National Organization for Rare Disorders. An organization dedicated to improving the lives of individuals and families living with a rare disease.

Nucleus ambiguus: A group of large motor neurons located deep in the medullary reticular formation; it innervates the muscles of the soft palate, pharynx, and larynx.

Odynophagia: The medical term for painful swallowing, experienced in the mouth, throat, or esophagus.

Organogenesis: The integrated process that changes cells into an organ during development of the embryo.

Osteopenia: A condition in which bone mineral density is lower than normal.

Palpebral fissure: The space separation between the margins of the upper and lower eyelids.

Paralysis: Complete loss of motor function and sensation of a given muscle group.

Paresis: Reduced ability in motor functioning of a muscle group with no concurrent loss of sensation.

Patellar reflex: A reflex contraction of the quadriceps muscle, resulting in a sudden involuntary extension of the leg.

Penetration: An event that occurs when food or liquid enters the trachea but stays above the level of the vocal folds; it is often a precursor to aspiration.

Percutaneous endoscopic gastrostomy (PEG) tube: An endoscopic medical procedure in which a tube is passed into the patient's stomach through the abdominal wall, most commonly to provide a means of feeding when oral intake is not adequate.

Pharynx: The membrane-lined cavity behind the nose and mouth, connecting them to the esophagus.

Phenotype: The set of observable characteristics of an individual resulting from the interaction of his or her genotype with the environment.

Pompe disease: An autosomal recessive, genetic disorder resulting in the buildup of glycogen in the cells of the body. This disorder is characterized by enlargement of the heart, progressive debilitation, organ failure, and death.

Pontocerebellar hypoplasia: A group of heterogenous neurodegenerative disorders with a prenatal onset affecting the cerebellum and pons. Common characteristics include atrophy of the cerebellum and pons, progressive microcephaly, and various cerebral involvement, including cognitive and motor impairments as well as seizures.

Ptosis: A drooping or falling of the upper eyelid.

Schwartz-Jampel syndrome: A rare genetic condition characterized by abnormalities of the skeletal muscles and bones.

Scoliosis: Abnormal lateral curvature of the spine.

Sequential Oral Sensory (SOS): A transdisciplinary feeding approach that integrates motor, oral, behavioral/learning, medical, sensory, and nutritional factors and approaches in order to comprehensively evaluate and manage children with feeding/growth problems.

Sideropenia: Iron deficiency in the blood serum.

Sphingomyelin: A type of sphingolipid found in animal cell membranes, especially in the membranous myelin sheath that surrounds some nerve cell axons.

Sporadic inclusion body myositis (sIBM): An acquired, progressive muscle disorder that becomes apparent during adulthood, characterized by progressive weakness and degeneration of the muscles of the arms and legs.

Stenosis: A narrowing of the space of a structure.

Stüve-Weidemann syndrome: A rare, autosomal recessive, congenital primary skeletal dysplasia, characterized by small stature, bowing of the long bones, camptodactyly, hyperthermic episodes, respiratory distress/apneic episodes, and feeding difficulty.

Thyroiditis: A general term that refers to inflammation of the thyroid gland.

Tracheoesophageal fistula: An abnormal connection in one or more places between the esophagus and the trachea.

Ulcer: A break in the lining of the stomach or duodenum that causes pain due to exposure to gastric acids.

VACTERL: An acronym for vertebral defects, anal atresia, cardiac defects, tracheo-esophageal fistula, renal anomalies, and limb abnormalities. Individuals diagnosed with VACTERL association typically have at least three of these characteristic features.

Wallenberg syndrome: A rare condition in which an infarction occurs in the lateral medulla, reducing the flow of oxygenated blood to this part of the brain and placing the individual at risk of stroke.

Zenker's diverticulum: Also known as a hypopharyngeal diverticulum; a pouch that can form at the junction of the hypopharynx and the esophagus.

Index

Note: Page numbers in **bold** reference non-text material.